Daily Meditation Tracker LogBook

This logbook belongs to

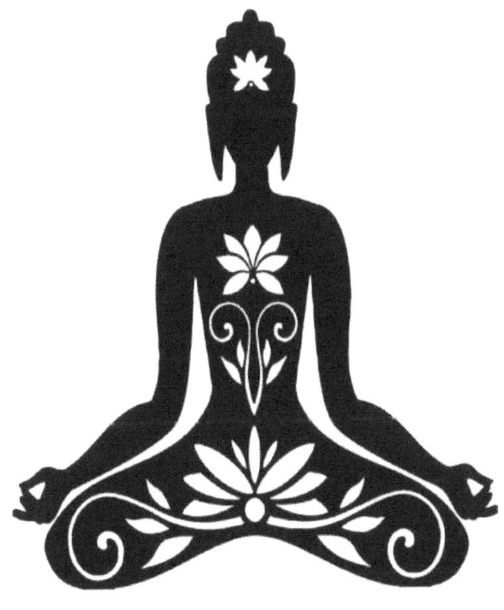

Personal Data

Name : _______________________________

Phone : _______________________________

Address : _______________________________

____

Incase of Emergency
Please Contact

Name : _______________________________

Phone : _______________________________

Address : _______________________________

____

Essential Contacts

Doctor : _______________________________

Pharmacy : _______________________________

Eye Clinic : _______________________________

Dentist : _______________________________

Name : _________________	Name : _________________
Call : _________________	Call : _________________
Work : _________________	Work : _________________
Home : _________________	Home : _________________
Email : _________________	Email : _________________
Other : _________________	Other : _________________
Name : _________________	Name : _________________
Call : _________________	Call : _________________
Work : _________________	Work : _________________
Home : _________________	Home : _________________
Email : _________________	Email : _________________
Other : _________________	Other : _________________

MEDITATION POSITION

MEDITATION FOCUS

MOOD WHEEL

THOUGHTS & INSIGHTS

QUALITY AND INTENSITY

FOCUS AND BREATHING

1 — 2 — 3 — 4 — 5 — 6 — 7 — 8 — 9 — 10

VISIONS AND EMOTIONS

REFLECTIONS

I am grateful for ...

I will accomplish ...

I need to work on ...

Notes

WHAT I LIKED

WHAT I DID NOT LIKE

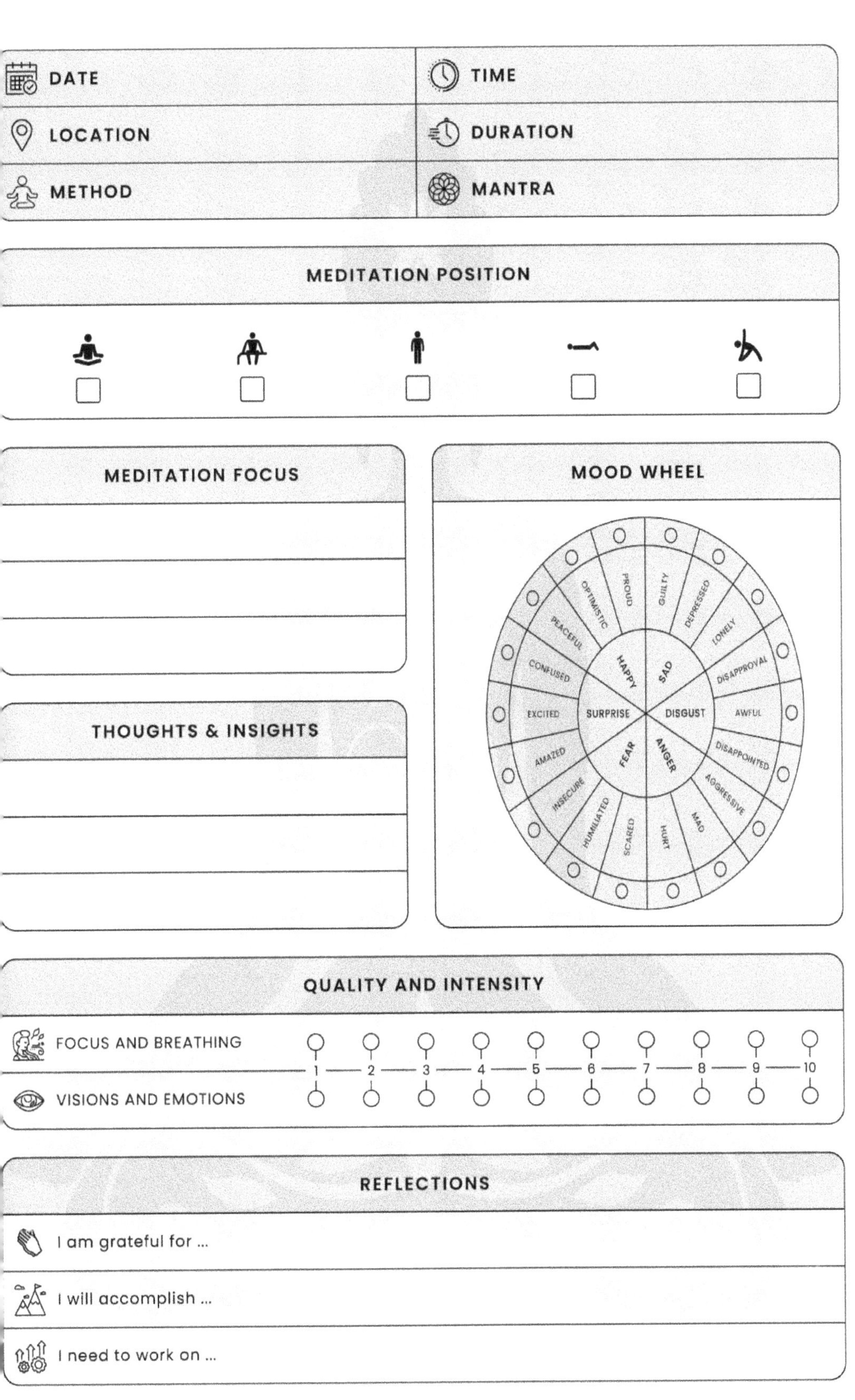

DATE	TIME
LOCATION	DURATION
METHOD	MANTRA

MEDITATION POSITION

☐ ☐ ☐ ☐ ☐

MEDITATION FOCUS

THOUGHTS & INSIGHTS

MOOD WHEEL

QUALITY AND INTENSITY

FOCUS AND BREATHING

1 — 2 — 3 — 4 — 5 — 6 — 7 — 8 — 9 — 10

VISIONS AND EMOTIONS

REFLECTIONS

I am grateful for ...

I will accomplish ...

I need to work on ...

Notes

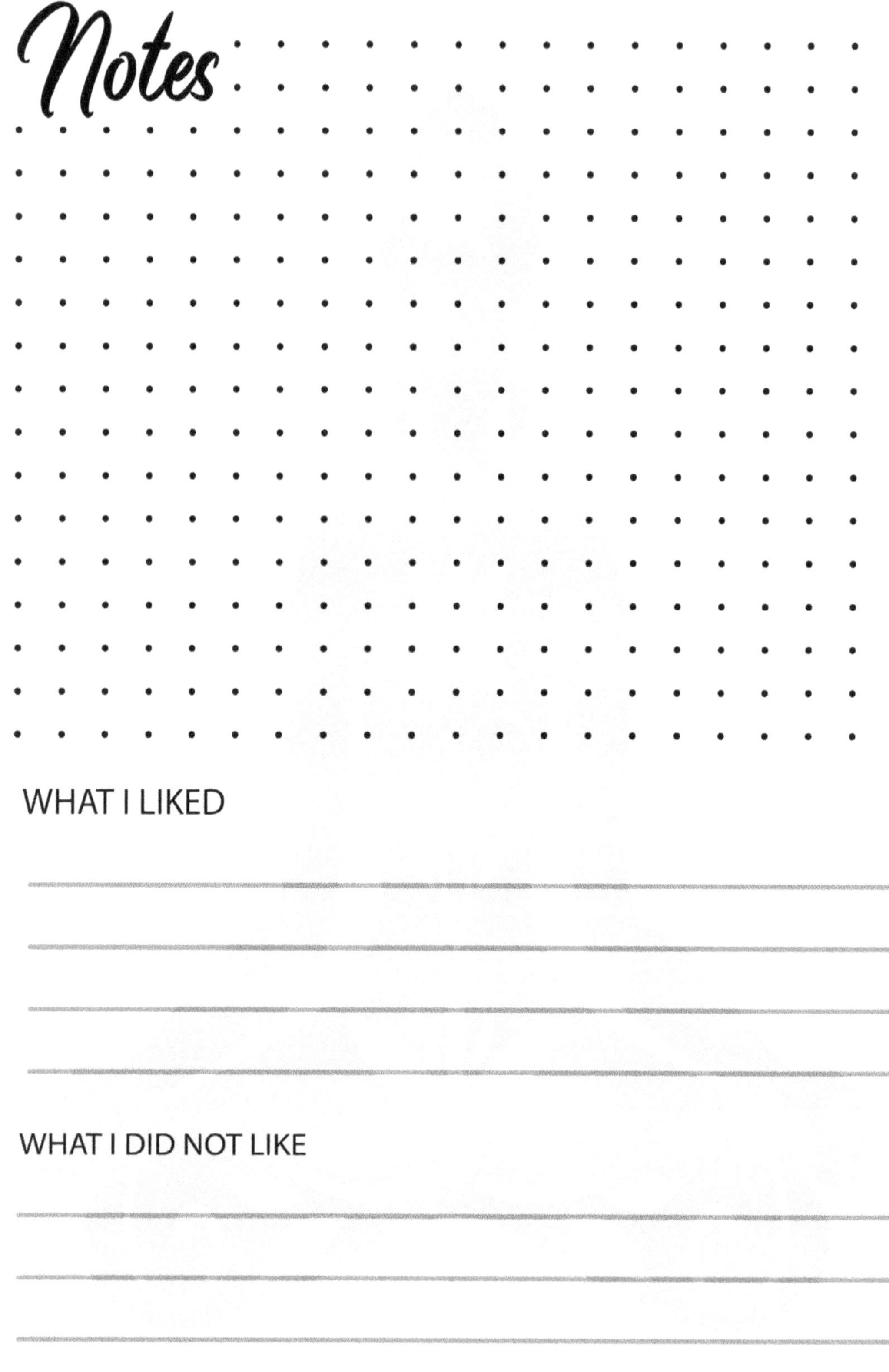

WHAT I LIKED

WHAT I DID NOT LIKE

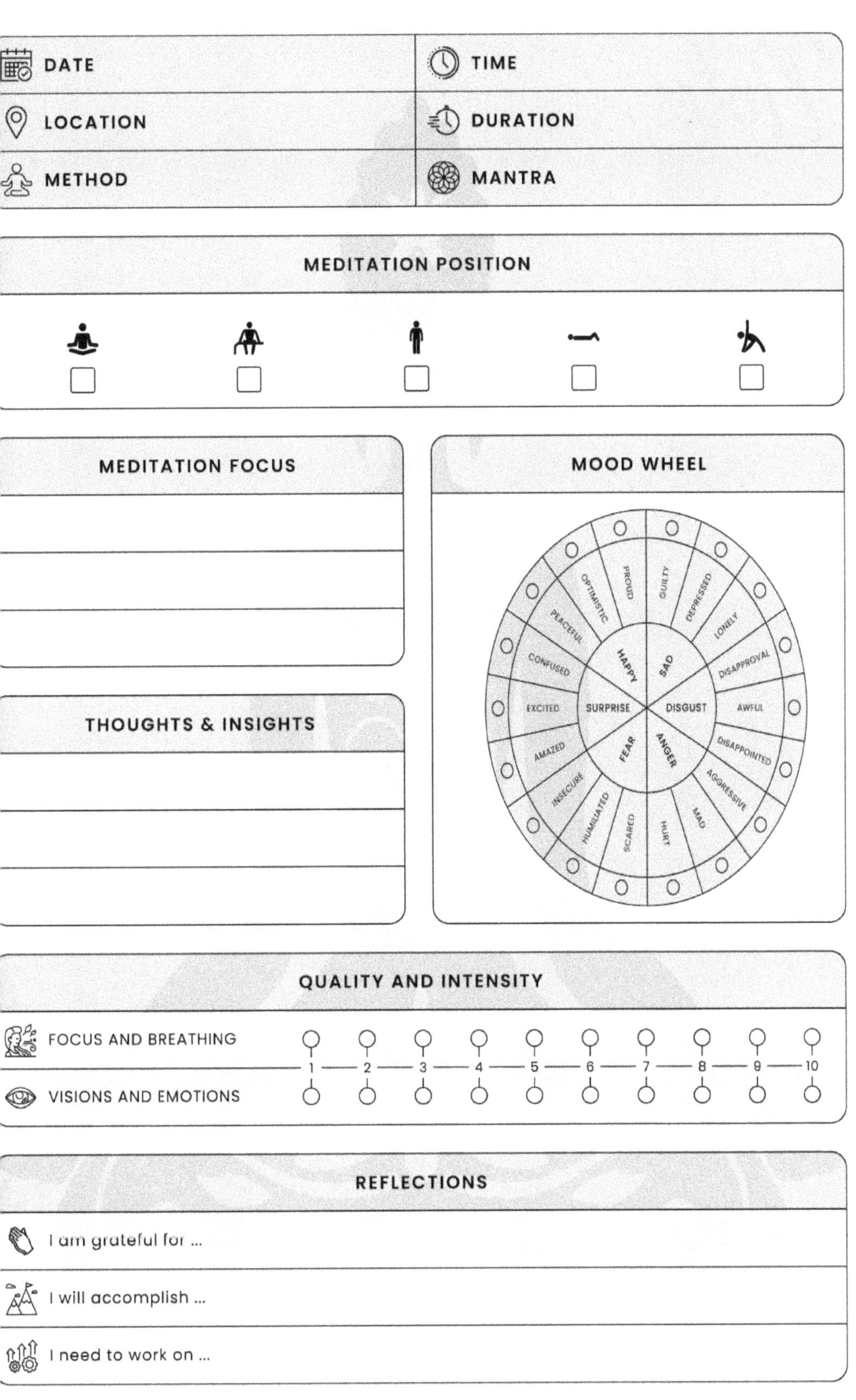

DATE	TIME
LOCATION	DURATION
METHOD	MANTRA

MEDITATION POSITION

☐ ☐ ☐ ☐ ☐

MEDITATION FOCUS

THOUGHTS & INSIGHTS

MOOD WHEEL

QUALITY AND INTENSITY

	1	2	3	4	5	6	7	8	9	10
FOCUS AND BREATHING	○	○	○	○	○	○	○	○	○	○
VISIONS AND EMOTIONS	○	○	○	○	○	○	○	○	○	○

REFLECTIONS

I am grateful for …

I will accomplish …

I need to work on …

Notes

WHAT I LIKED

WHAT I DID NOT LIKE

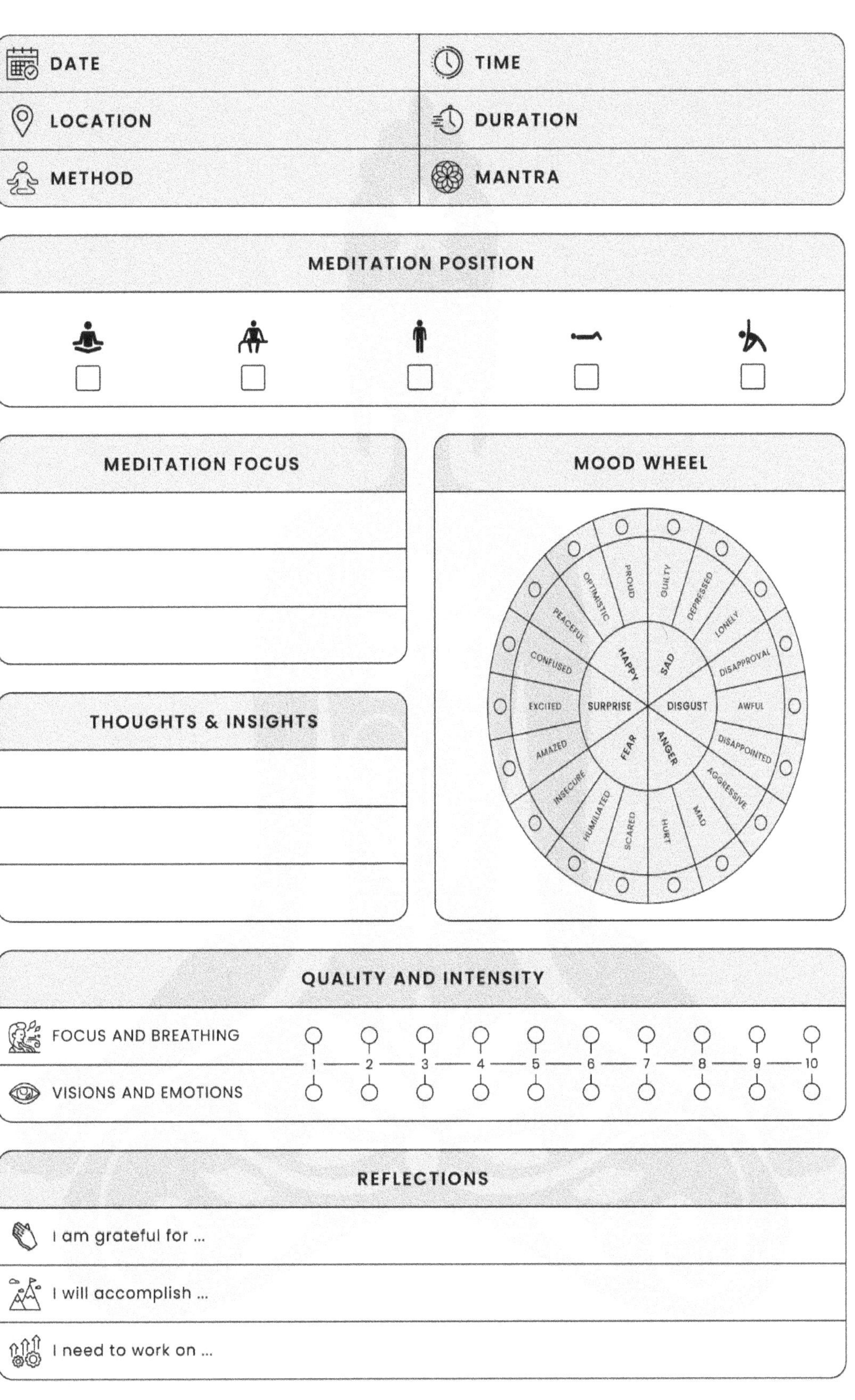

DATE
TIME
LOCATION
DURATION
METHOD
MANTRA

MEDITATION POSITION

MEDITATION FOCUS

MOOD WHEEL

OPTIMISTIC
PROUD
GUILTY
DEPRESSED
PEACEFUL
LONELY
CONFUSED
DISAPPROVAL
HAPPY
SAD
EXCITED
SURPRISE
DISGUST
AWFUL
AMAZED
FEAR
ANGER
DISAPPOINTED
INSECURE
AGGRESSIVE
HUMILIATED
SCARED
HURT
MAD

THOUGHTS & INSIGHTS

QUALITY AND INTENSITY

FOCUS AND BREATHING
1 — 2 — 3 — 4 — 5 — 6 — 7 — 8 — 9 — 10
VISIONS AND EMOTIONS

REFLECTIONS

I am grateful for ...
I will accomplish ...
I need to work on ...

Notes

WHAT I LIKED

WHAT I DID NOT LIKE

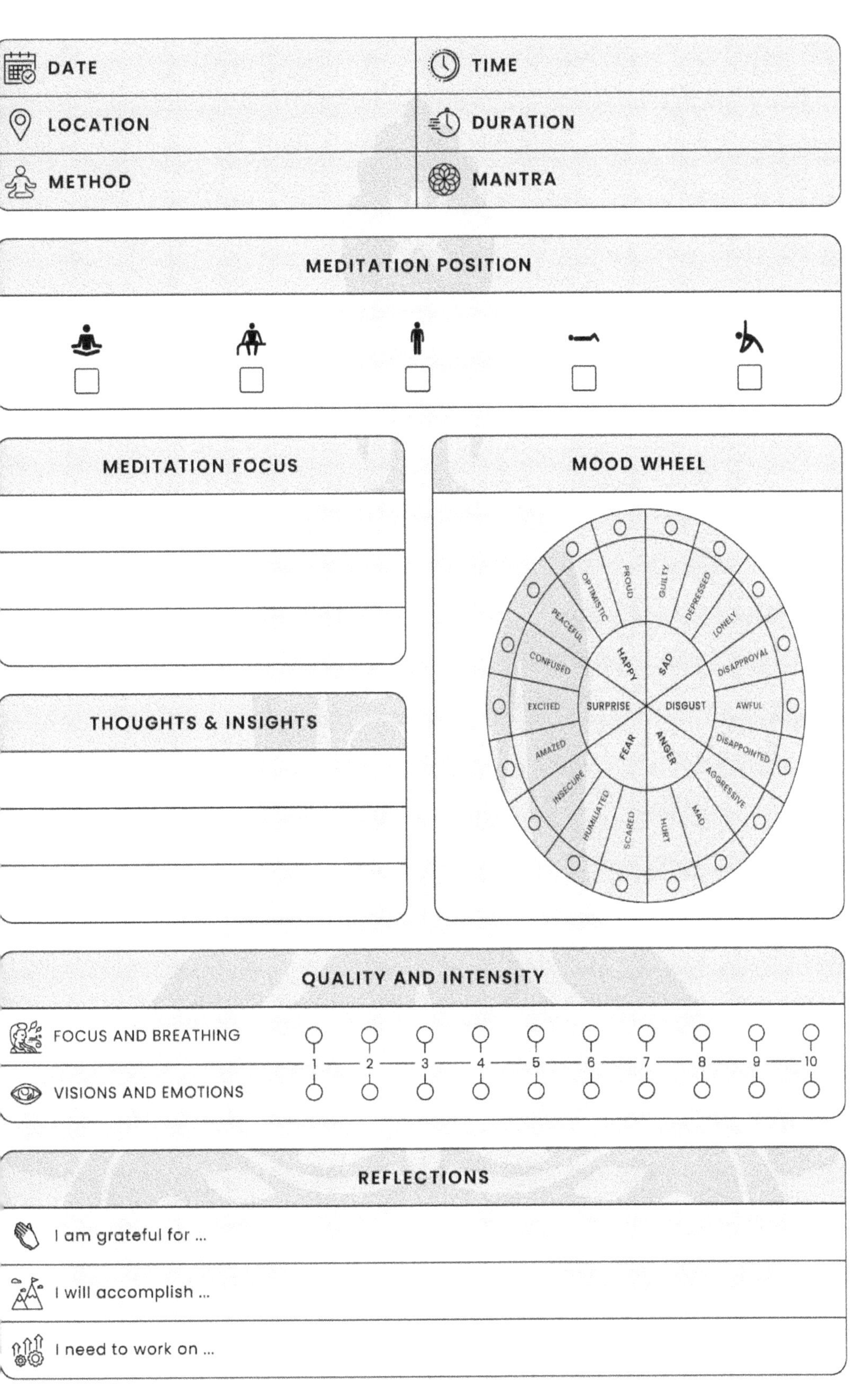

DATE
TIME
LOCATION
DURATION
METHOD
MANTRA

MEDITATION POSITION

MEDITATION FOCUS

THOUGHTS & INSIGHTS

MOOD WHEEL

OPTIMISTIC
PROUD
GUILTY
DEPRESSED
PEACEFUL
LONELY
CONFUSED
HAPPY
SAD
DISAPPROVAL
EXCITED
SURPRISE
DISGUST
AWFUL
AMAZED
FEAR
ANGER
DISAPPOINTED
INSECURE
AGGRESSIVE
HUMILIATED
SCARED
HURT
MAD

QUALITY AND INTENSITY

FOCUS AND BREATHING
1 — 2 — 3 — 4 — 5 — 6 — 7 — 8 — 9 — 10
VISIONS AND EMOTIONS

REFLECTIONS

I am grateful for ...

I will accomplish ...

I need to work on ...

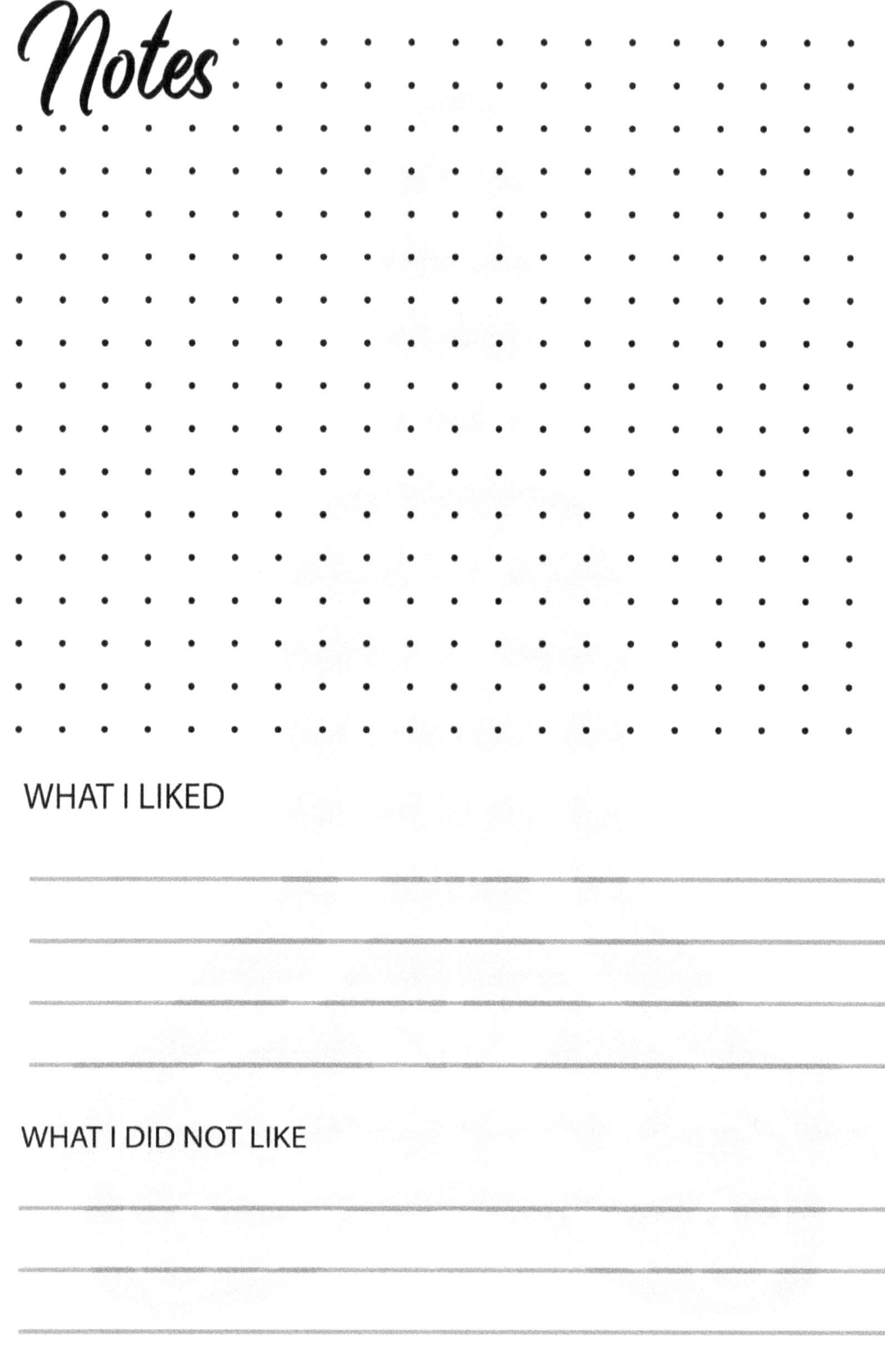

Notes

WHAT I LIKED

WHAT I DID NOT LIKE

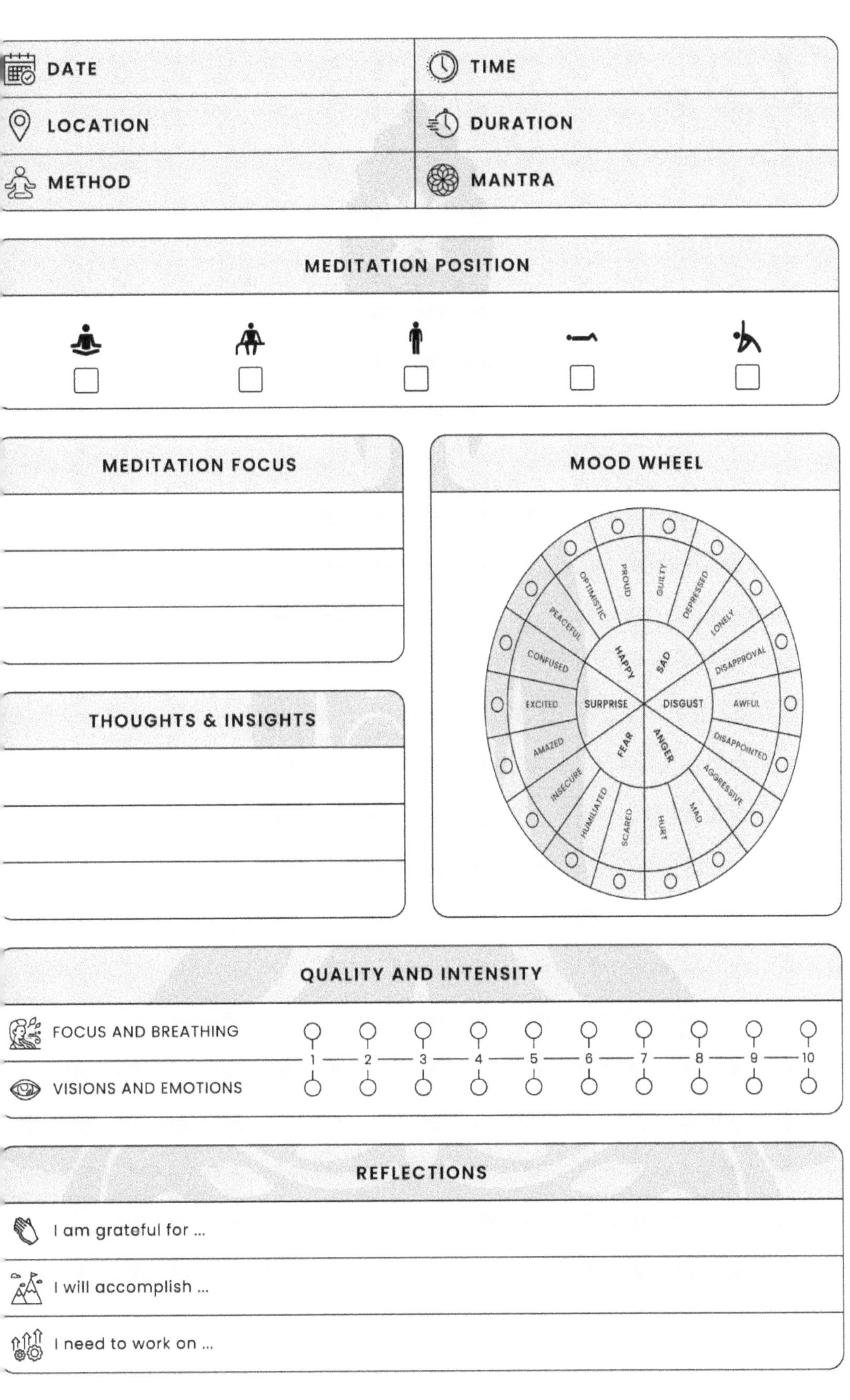

DATE
TIME
LOCATION
DURATION
METHOD
MANTRA

MEDITATION POSITION

MEDITATION FOCUS

MOOD WHEEL

OPTIMISTIC
PROUD
GUILTY
DEPRESSED
PEACEFUL
LONELY
CONFUSED
DISAPPROVAL
HAPPY
SAD
EXCITED
SURPRISE
DISGUST
AWFUL
AMAZED
FEAR
ANGER
DISAPPOINTED
INSECURE
AGGRESSIVE
HUMILIATED
SCARED
HURT
MAD

THOUGHTS & INSIGHTS

QUALITY AND INTENSITY

FOCUS AND BREATHING
1 — 2 — 3 — 4 — 5 — 6 — 7 — 8 — 9 — 10
VISIONS AND EMOTIONS

REFLECTIONS

I am grateful for ...

I will accomplish ...

I need to work on ...

Notes

WHAT I LIKED

WHAT I DID NOT LIKE

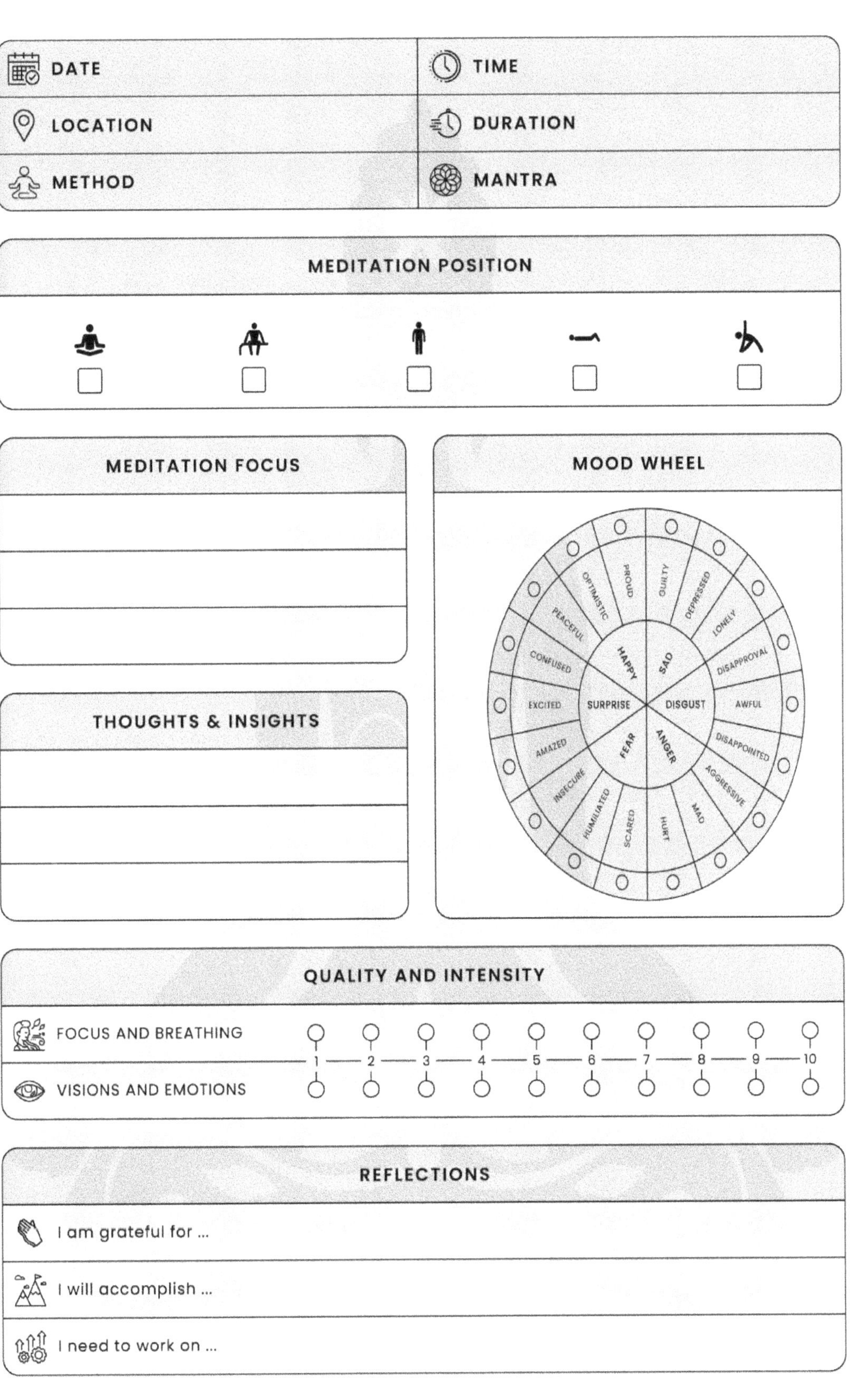

DATE
TIME
LOCATION
DURATION
METHOD
MANTRA
MEDITATION POSITION
MEDITATION FOCUS
MOOD WHEEL
OPTIMISTIC
PROUD
GUILTY
DEPRESSED
PEACEFUL
LONELY
CONFUSED
DISAPPROVAL
HAPPY
SAD
EXCITED
SURPRISE
DISGUST
AWFUL
AMAZED
FEAR
ANGER
DISAPPOINTED
INSECURE
AGGRESSIVE
HUMILIATED
SCARED
HURT
MAD
THOUGHTS & INSIGHTS
QUALITY AND INTENSITY
FOCUS AND BREATHING
1 — 2 — 3 — 4 — 5 — 6 — 7 — 8 — 9 — 10
VISIONS AND EMOTIONS
REFLECTIONS
I am grateful for ...
I will accomplish ...
I need to work on ...

Notes

WHAT I LIKED

WHAT I DID NOT LIKE

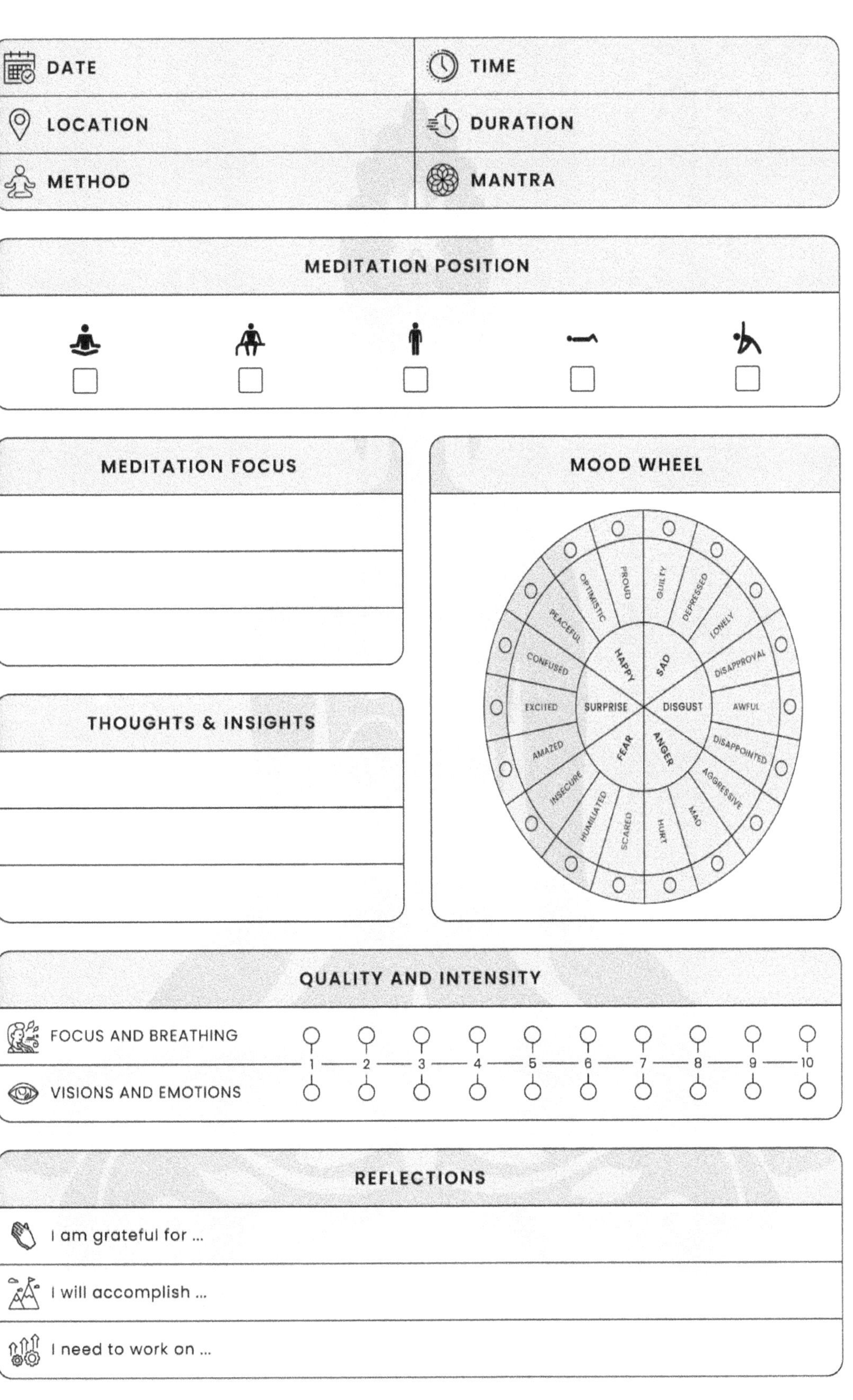

DATE
TIME
LOCATION
DURATION
METHOD
MANTRA

MEDITATION POSITION

MEDITATION FOCUS

MOOD WHEEL

OPTIMISTIC
PROUD
GUILTY
DEPRESSED
PEACEFUL
LONELY
CONFUSED
DISAPPROVAL
HAPPY
SAD
EXCITED
SURPRISE
DISGUST
AWFUL
AMAZED
FEAR
ANGER
DISAPPOINTED
INSECURE
AGGRESSIVE
HUMILIATED
MAD
SCARED
HURT

THOUGHTS & INSIGHTS

QUALITY AND INTENSITY

FOCUS AND BREATHING
1 — 2 — 3 — 4 — 5 — 6 — 7 — 8 — 9 — 10
VISIONS AND EMOTIONS

REFLECTIONS

I am grateful for ...

I will accomplish ...

I need to work on ...

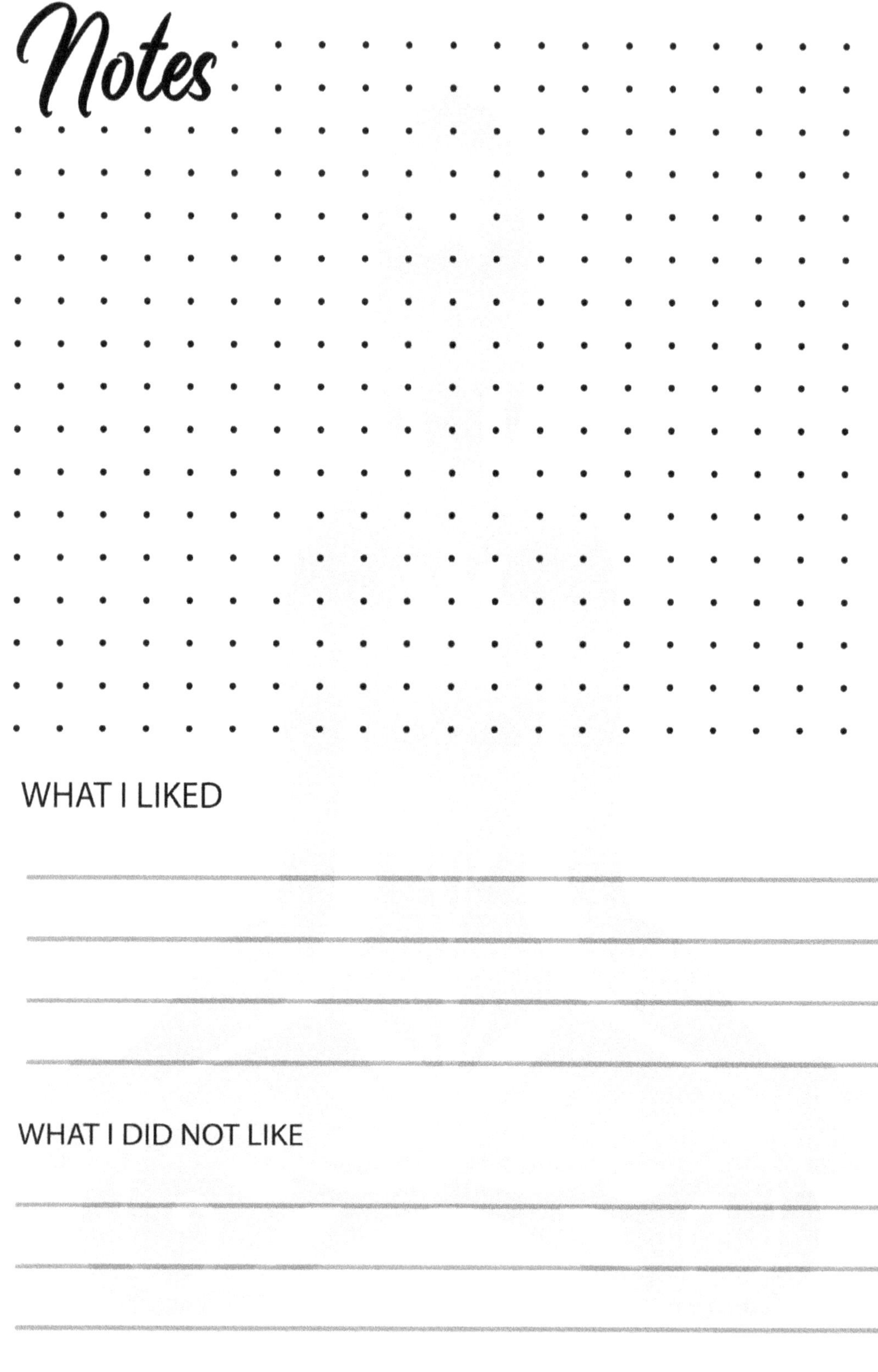

Notes

WHAT I LIKED

WHAT I DID NOT LIKE

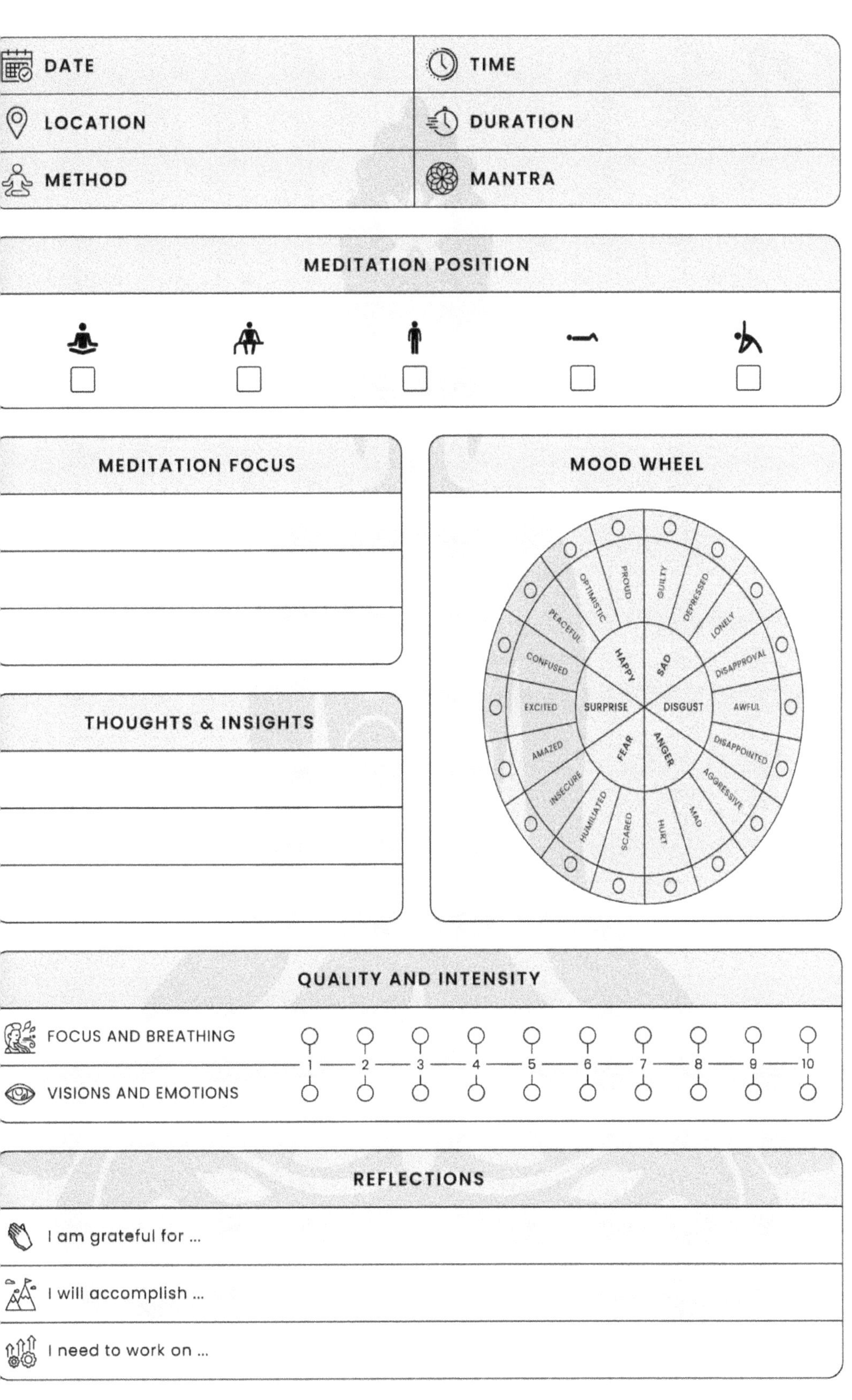

DATE
TIME
LOCATION
DURATION
METHOD
MANTRA

MEDITATION POSITION

MEDITATION FOCUS

MOOD WHEEL

OPTIMISTIC
PROUD
GUILTY
DEPRESSED
PEACEFUL
LONELY
CONFUSED
DISAPPROVAL
HAPPY
SAD
EXCITED
SURPRISE
DISGUST
AWFUL
AMAZED
FEAR
ANGER
DISAPPOINTED
INSECURE
AGGRESSIVE
HUMILIATED
SCARED
HURT
MAD

THOUGHTS & INSIGHTS

QUALITY AND INTENSITY

FOCUS AND BREATHING
1 — 2 — 3 — 4 — 5 — 6 — 7 — 8 — 9 — 10
VISIONS AND EMOTIONS

REFLECTIONS

I am grateful for ...

I will accomplish ...

I need to work on ...

Notes

WHAT I LIKED

WHAT I DID NOT LIKE

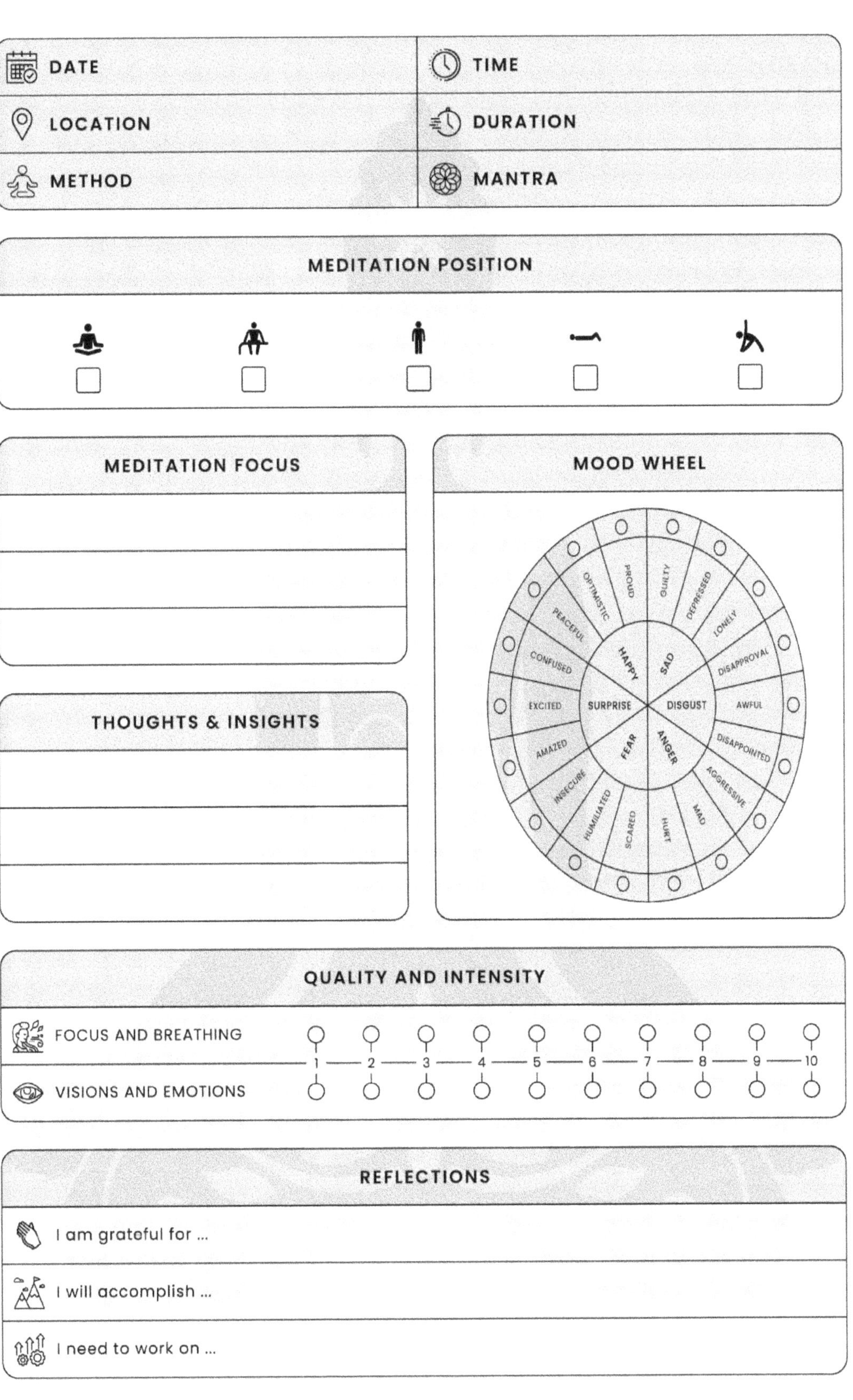

DATE
TIME
LOCATION
DURATION
METHOD
MANTRA
MEDITATION POSITION
MEDITATION FOCUS
MOOD WHEEL
OPTIMISTIC
PROUD
GUILTY
DEPRESSED
PEACEFUL
LONELY
CONFUSED
HAPPY
SAD
DISAPPROVAL
EXCITED
SURPRISE
DISGUST
AWFUL
AMAZED
FEAR
ANGER
DISAPPOINTED
INSECURE
AGGRESSIVE
HUMILIATED
SCARED
HURT
MAD
THOUGHTS & INSIGHTS
QUALITY AND INTENSITY
FOCUS AND BREATHING
1 — 2 — 3 — 4 — 5 — 6 — 7 — 8 — 9 — 10
VISIONS AND EMOTIONS
REFLECTIONS
I am grateful for ...
I will accomplish ...
I need to work on ...

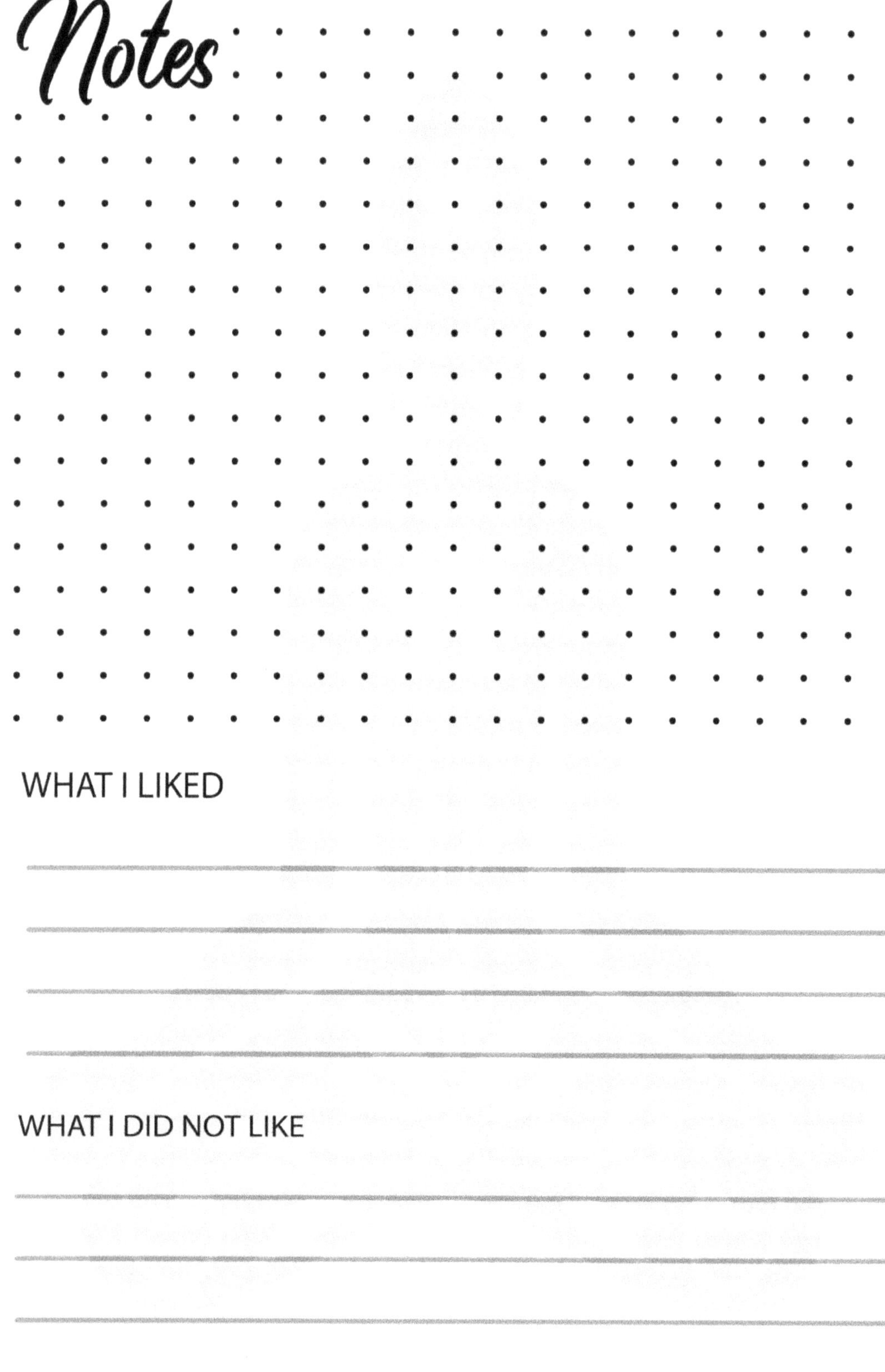# Notes

WHAT I LIKED

WHAT I DID NOT LIKE

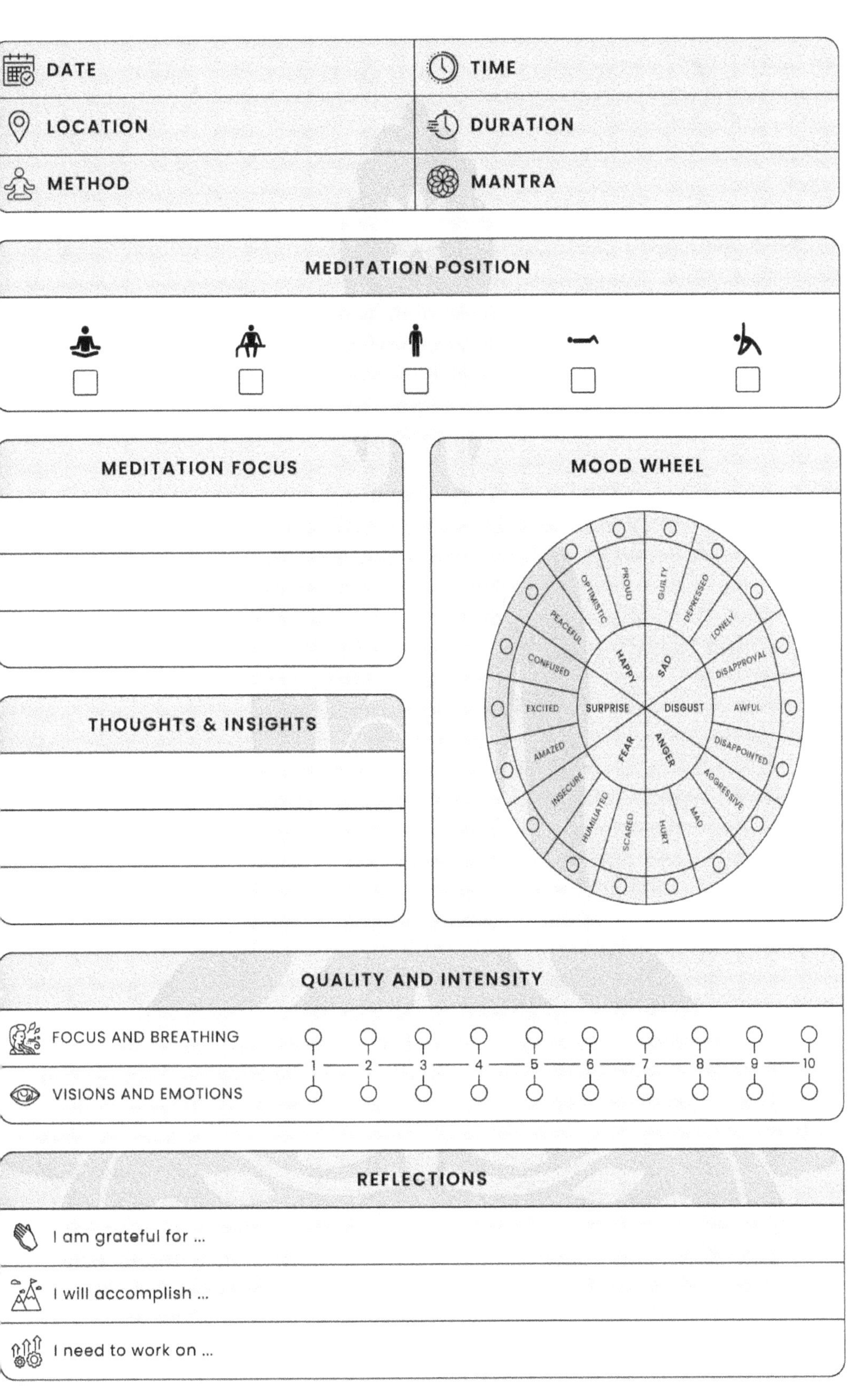

DATE
TIME
LOCATION
DURATION
METHOD
MANTRA
MEDITATION POSITION
MEDITATION FOCUS
MOOD WHEEL
OPTIMISTIC
PROUD
GUILTY
DEPRESSED
PEACEFUL
LONELY
CONFUSED
HAPPY
SAD
DISAPPROVAL
EXCITED
SURPRISE
DISGUST
AWFUL
AMAZED
FEAR
ANGER
DISAPPOINTED
INSECURE
AGGRESSIVE
HUMILIATED
SCARED
HURT
MAD
THOUGHTS & INSIGHTS
QUALITY AND INTENSITY
FOCUS AND BREATHING
1 2 3 4 5 6 7 8 9 10
VISIONS AND EMOTIONS
REFLECTIONS
I am grateful for ...
I will accomplish ...
I need to work on ...

Notes

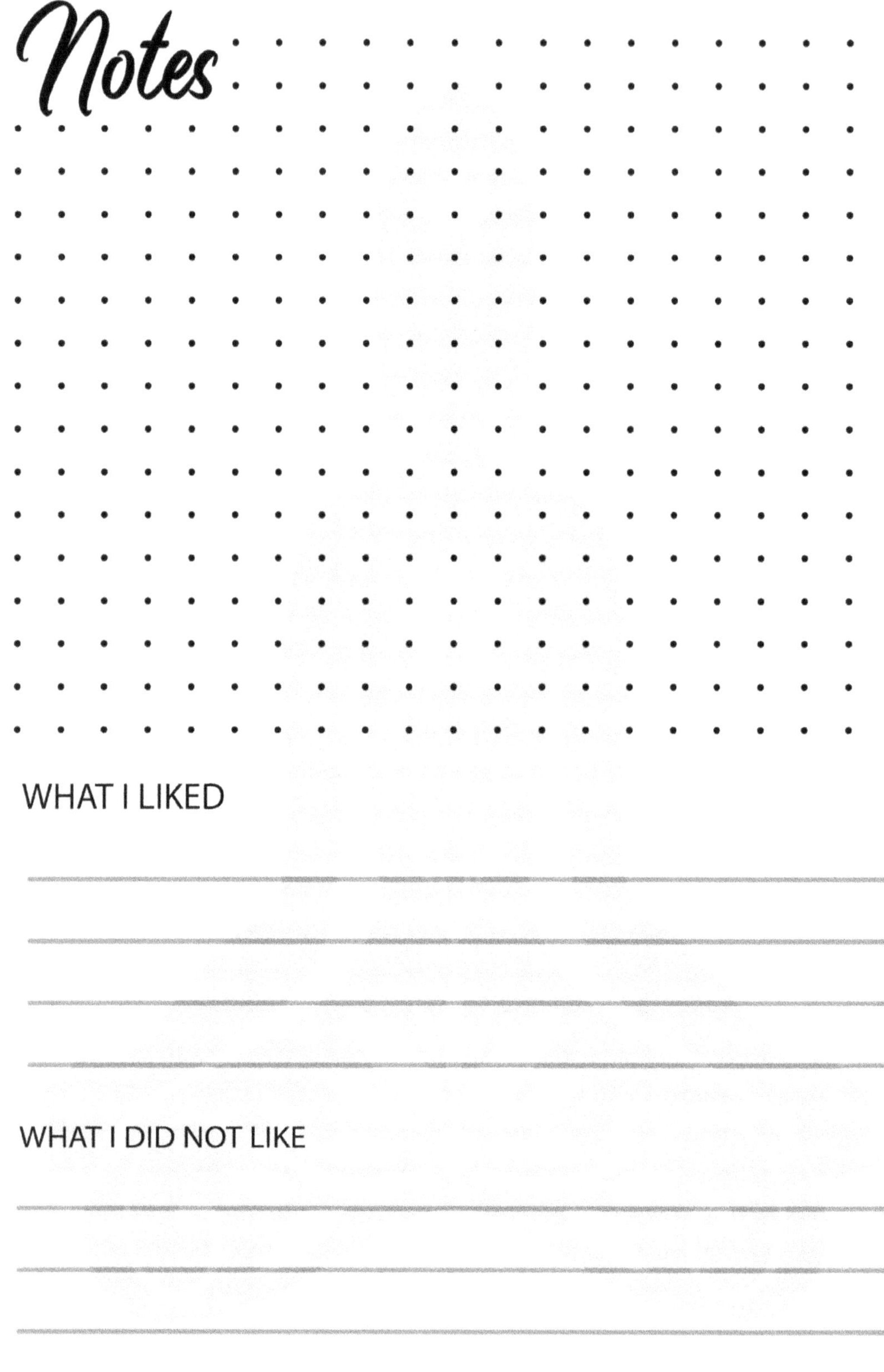

WHAT I LIKED

WHAT I DID NOT LIKE

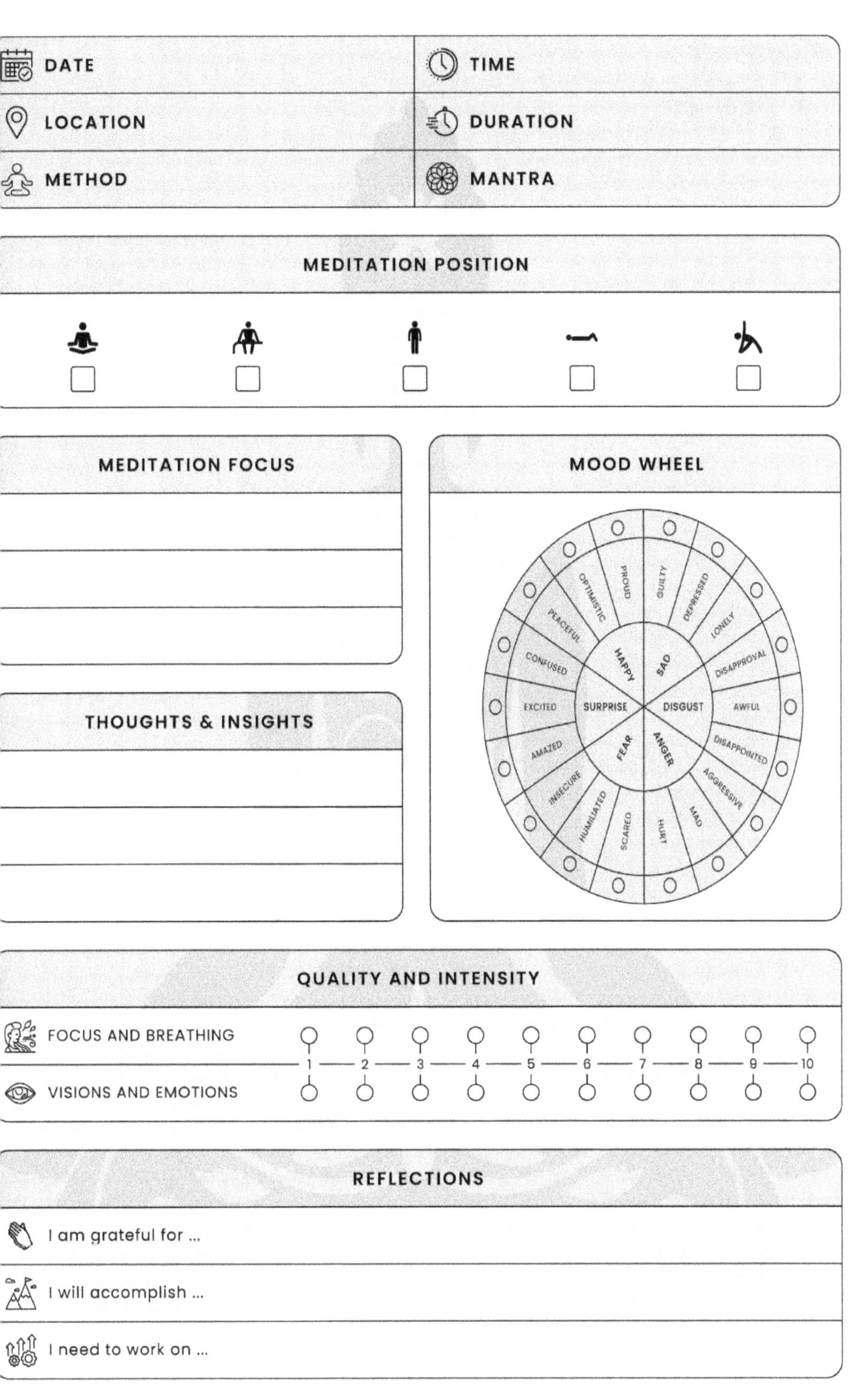

DATE
TIME
LOCATION
DURATION
METHOD
MANTRA
MEDITATION POSITION
MEDITATION FOCUS
MOOD WHEEL
OPTIMISTIC
PROUD
GUILTY
DEPRESSED
PEACEFUL
LONELY
CONFUSED
DISAPPROVAL
HAPPY
SAD
EXCITED
SURPRISE
DISGUST
AWFUL
AMAZED
FEAR
ANGER
DISAPPOINTED
INSECURE
AGGRESSIVE
HUMILIATED
SCARED
HURT
MAD
THOUGHTS & INSIGHTS
QUALITY AND INTENSITY
FOCUS AND BREATHING
1 2 3 4 5 6 7 8 9 10
VISIONS AND EMOTIONS
REFLECTIONS
I am grateful for ...
I will accomplish ...
I need to work on ...

Notes

WHAT I LIKED

WHAT I DID NOT LIKE

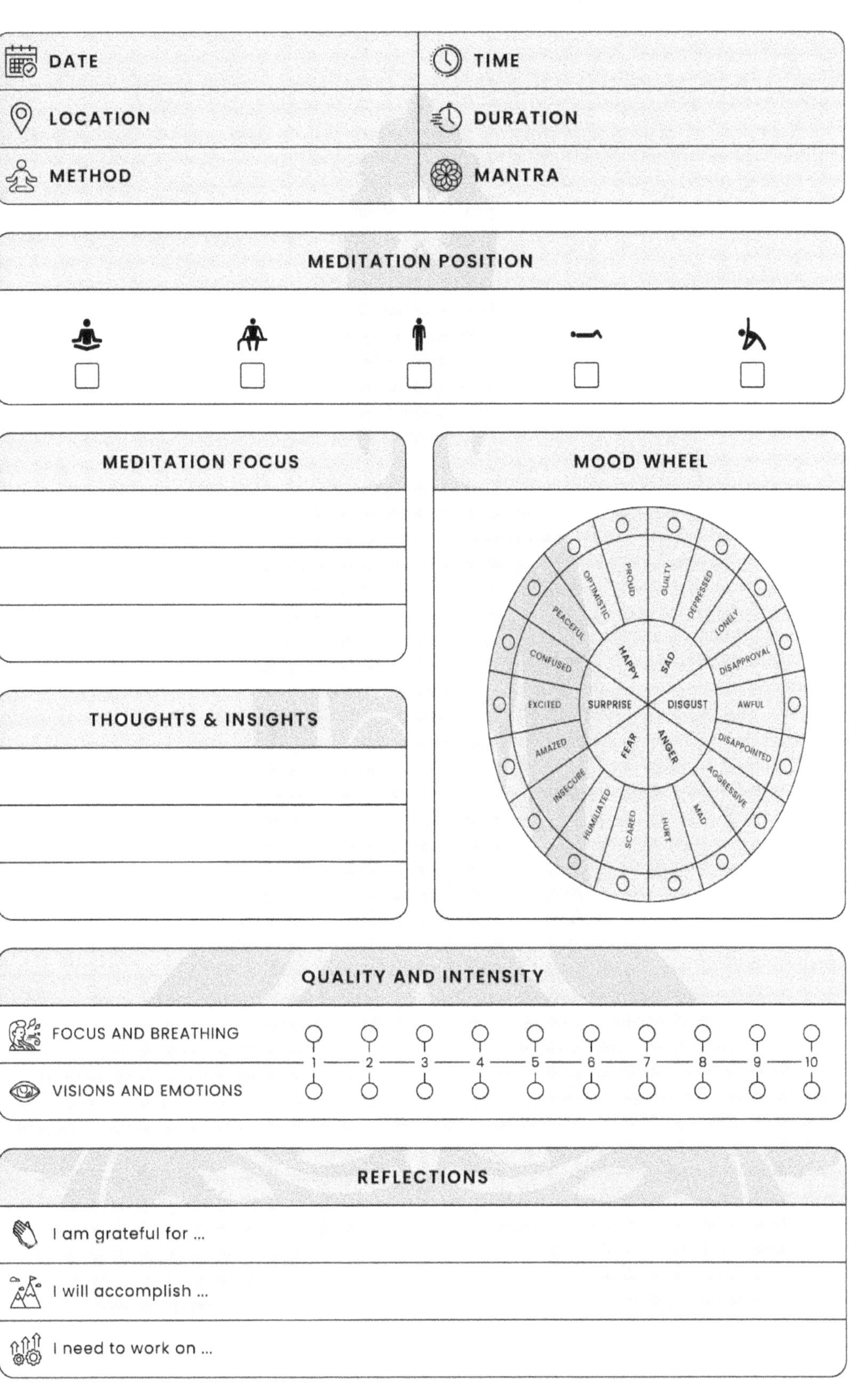

DATE
TIME
LOCATION
DURATION
METHOD
MANTRA
MEDITATION POSITION
MEDITATION FOCUS
MOOD WHEEL
OPTIMISTIC
PROUD
GUILTY
DEPRESSED
PEACEFUL
LONELY
CONFUSED
HAPPY
SAD
DISAPPROVAL
EXCITED
SURPRISE
DISGUST
AWFUL
AMAZED
FEAR
ANGER
DISAPPOINTED
INSECURE
AGGRESSIVE
HUMILIATED
SCARED
HURT
MAD
THOUGHTS & INSIGHTS
QUALITY AND INTENSITY
FOCUS AND BREATHING
1 2 3 4 5 6 7 8 9 10
VISIONS AND EMOTIONS
REFLECTIONS
I am grateful for ...
I will accomplish ...
I need to work on ...

Notes

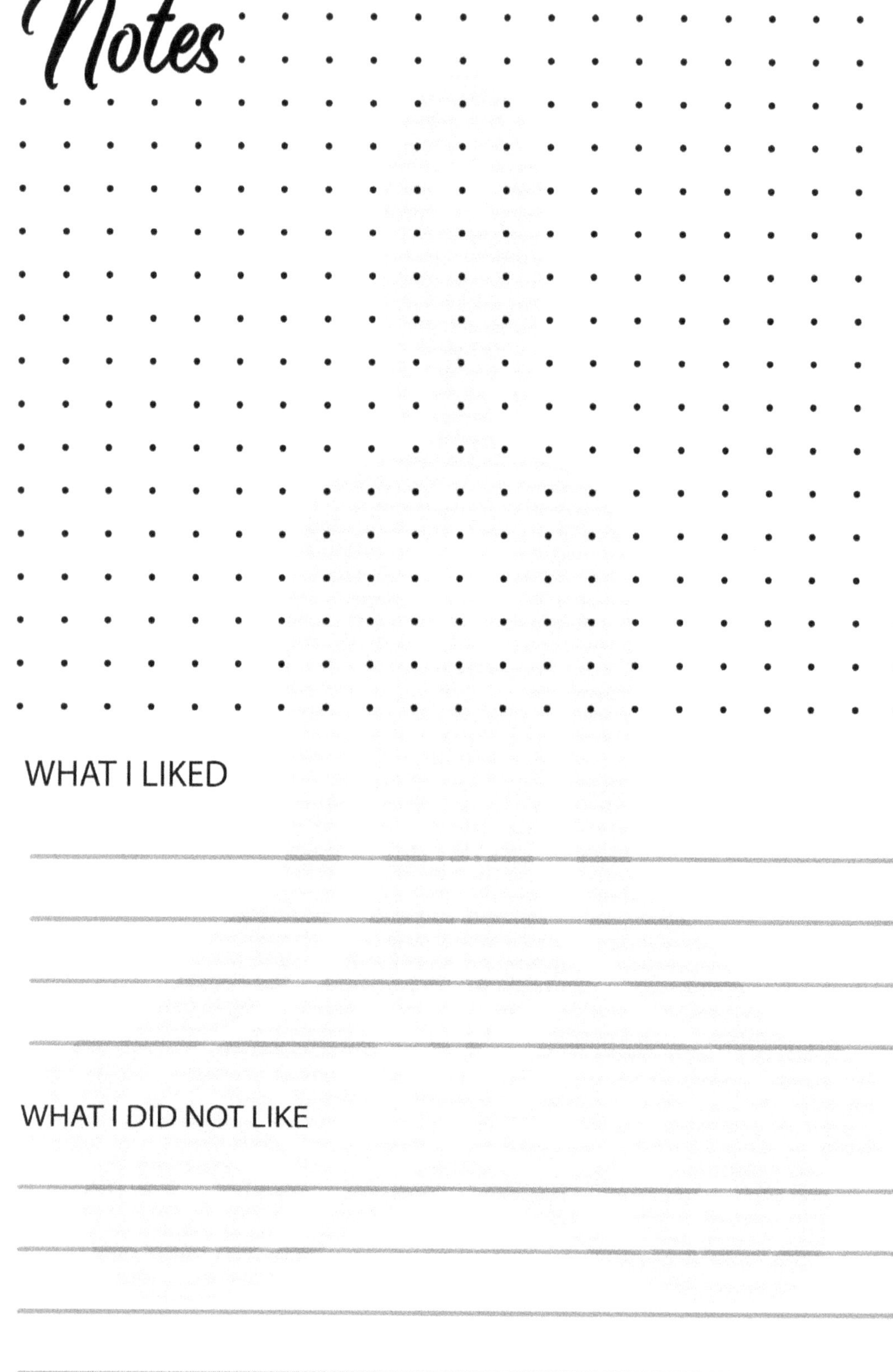

WHAT I LIKED

WHAT I DID NOT LIKE

MEDITATION POSITION

MEDITATION FOCUS

MOOD WHEEL

THOUGHTS & INSIGHTS

QUALITY AND INTENSITY

FOCUS AND BREATHING

1 — 2 — 3 — 4 — 5 — 6 — 7 — 8 — 9 — 10

VISIONS AND EMOTIONS

REFLECTIONS

I am grateful for ...

I will accomplish ...

I need to work on ...

Notes

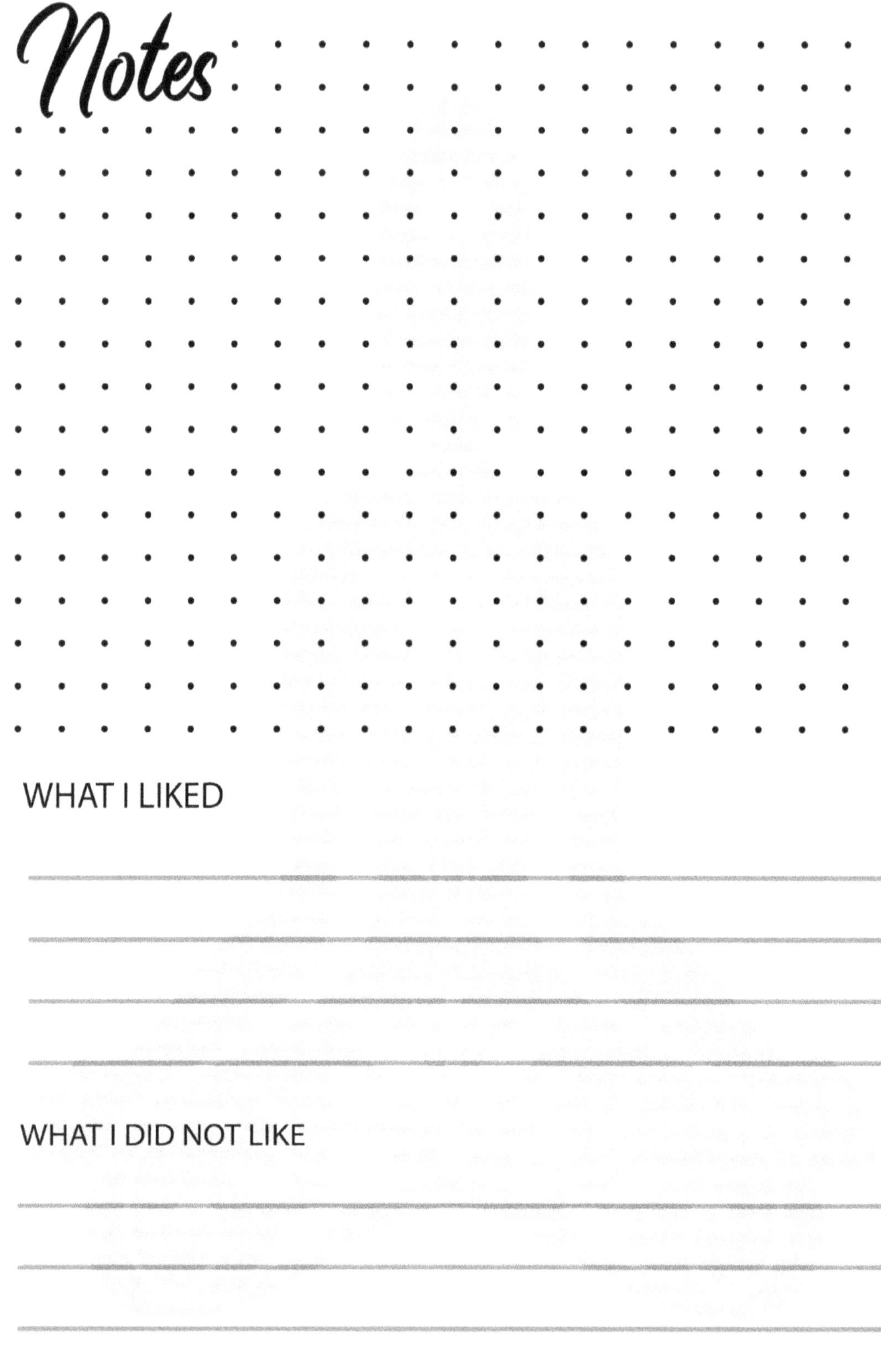

WHAT I LIKED

WHAT I DID NOT LIKE

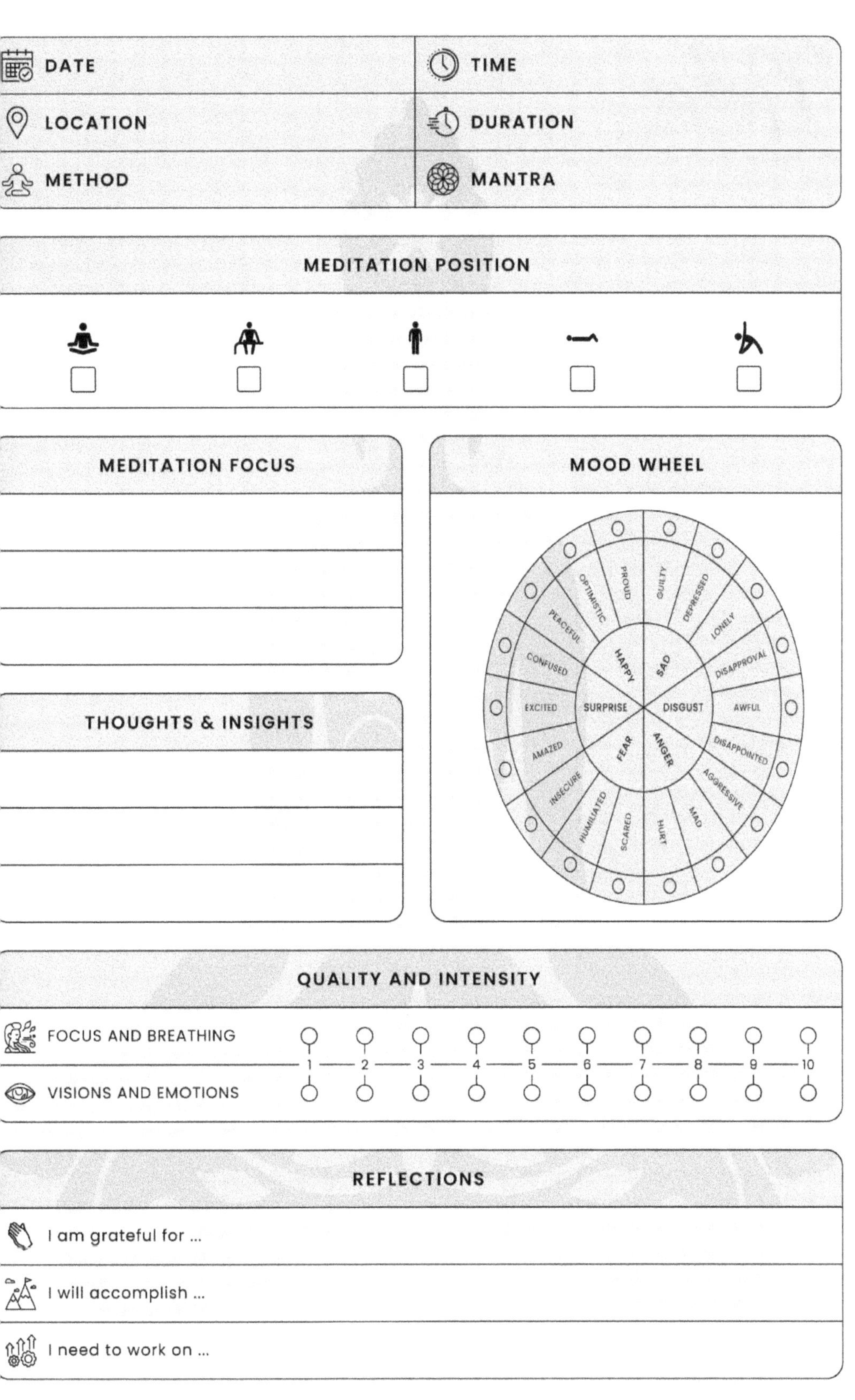

DATE
TIME
LOCATION
DURATION
METHOD
MANTRA
MEDITATION POSITION
MEDITATION FOCUS
MOOD WHEEL
OPTIMISTIC
PROUD
GUILTY
DEPRESSED
PEACEFUL
LONELY
CONFUSED
HAPPY
SAD
DISAPPROVAL
EXCITED
SURPRISE
DISGUST
AWFUL
AMAZED
FEAR
ANGER
DISAPPOINTED
INSECURE
AGGRESSIVE
HUMILIATED
SCARED
HURT
MAD
THOUGHTS & INSIGHTS
QUALITY AND INTENSITY
FOCUS AND BREATHING
1 2 3 4 5 6 7 8 9 10
VISIONS AND EMOTIONS
REFLECTIONS
I am grateful for ...
I will accomplish ...
I need to work on ...

Notes

WHAT I LIKED

WHAT I DID NOT LIKE

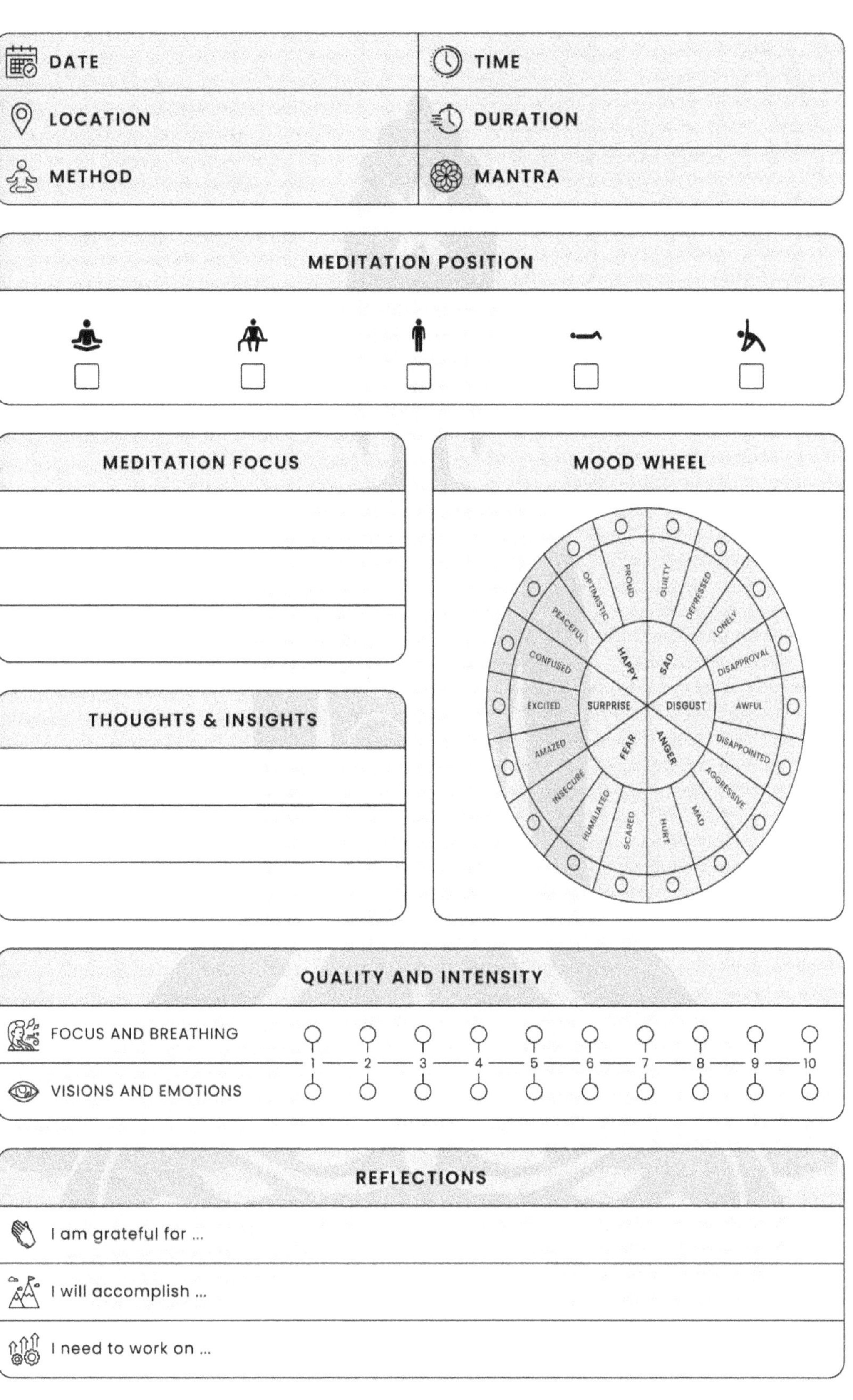

DATE
TIME
LOCATION
DURATION
METHOD
MANTRA

MEDITATION POSITION

MEDITATION FOCUS

MOOD WHEEL

OPTIMISTIC
PROUD
GUILTY
DEPRESSED
PEACEFUL
LONELY
CONFUSED
HAPPY
SAD
DISAPPROVAL
EXCITED
SURPRISE
DISGUST
AWFUL
AMAZED
FEAR
ANGER
DISAPPOINTED
INSECURE
AGGRESSIVE
HUMILIATED
SCARED
HURT
MAD

THOUGHTS & INSIGHTS

QUALITY AND INTENSITY

FOCUS AND BREATHING
1 — 2 — 3 — 4 — 5 — 6 — 7 — 8 — 9 — 10
VISIONS AND EMOTIONS

REFLECTIONS

I am grateful for ...

I will accomplish ...

I need to work on ...

Notes

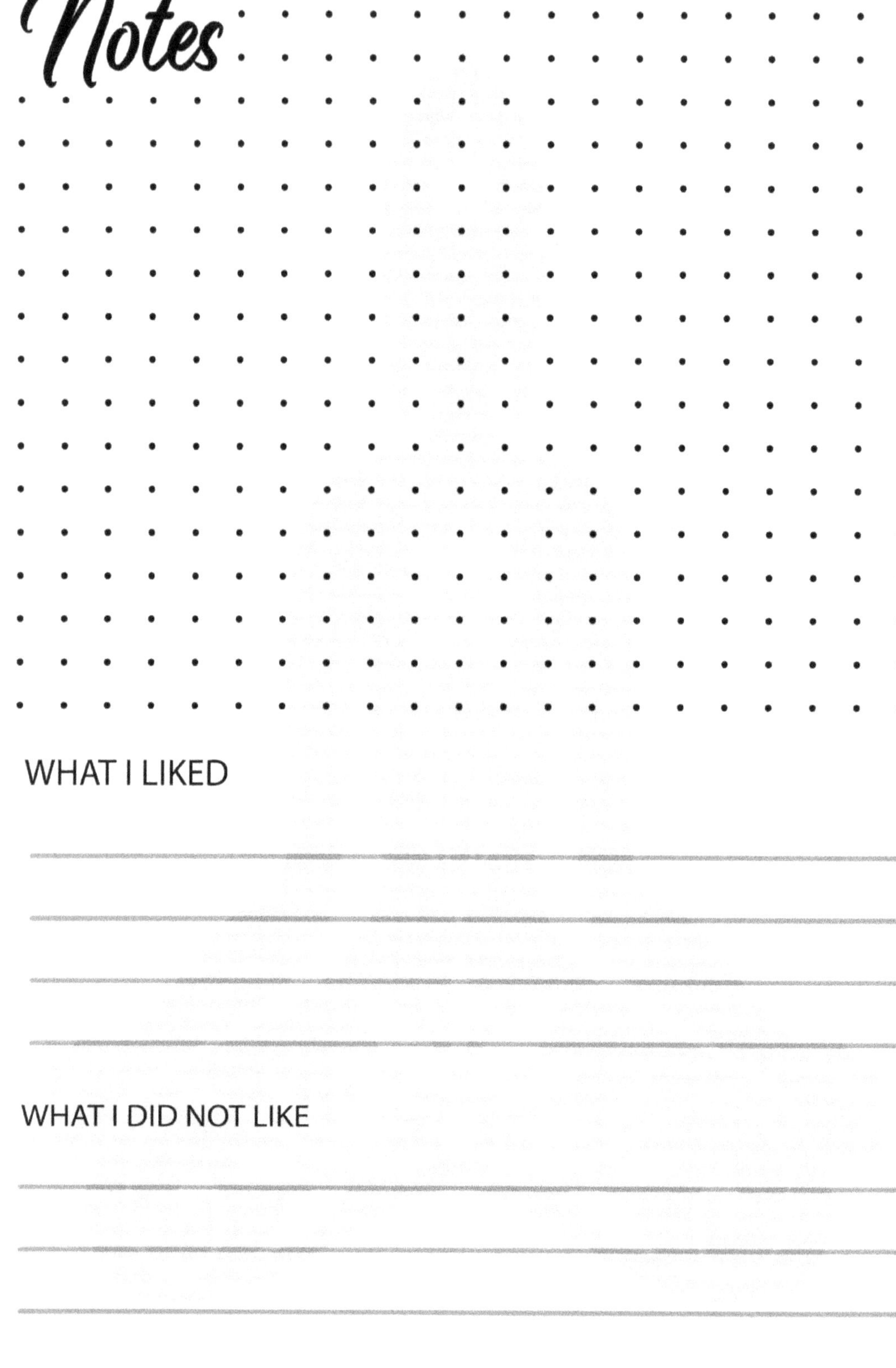

WHAT I LIKED

WHAT I DID NOT LIKE

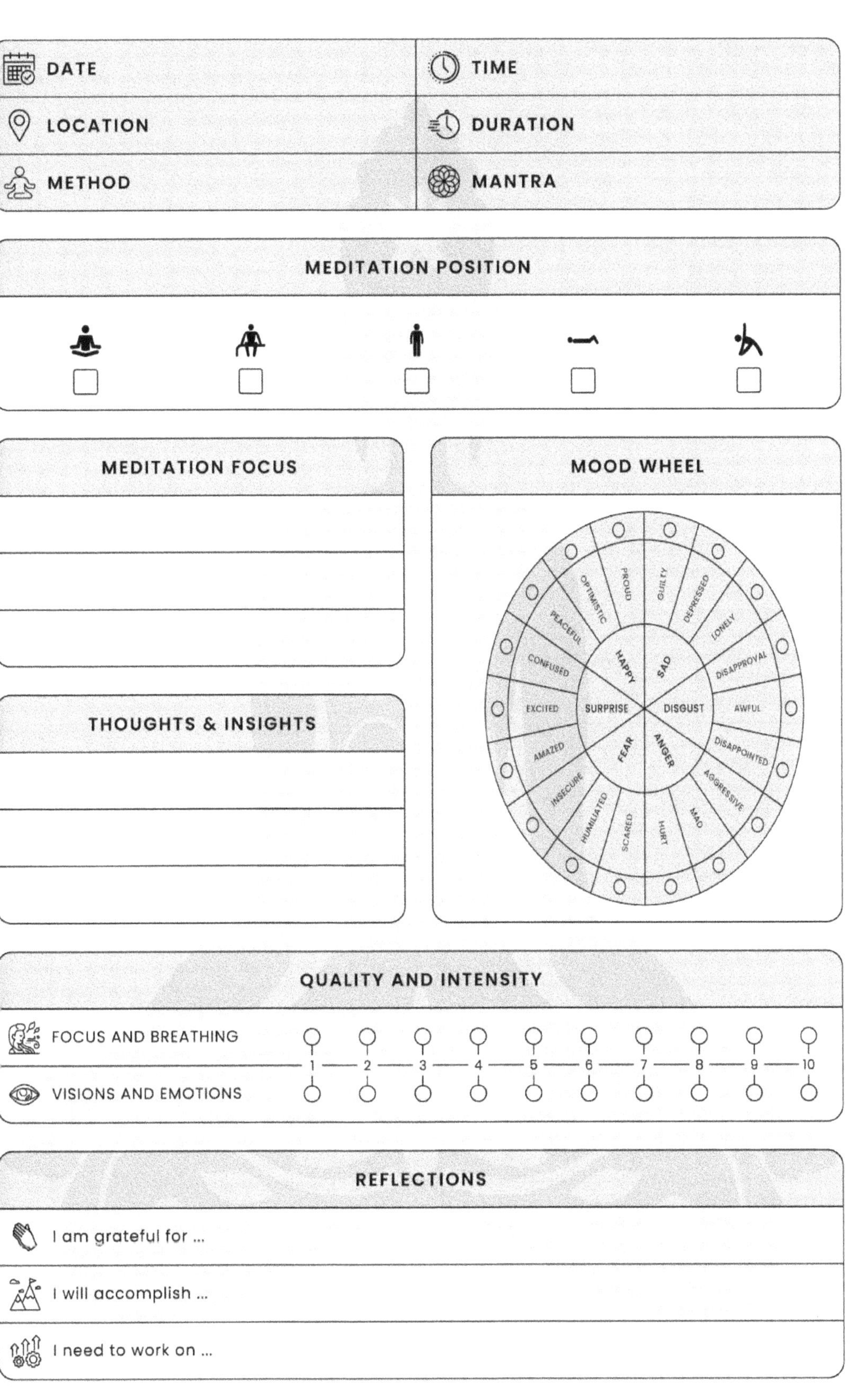

DATE
TIME
LOCATION
DURATION
METHOD
MANTRA
MEDITATION POSITION
MEDITATION FOCUS
MOOD WHEEL
OPTIMISTIC
PROUD
GUILTY
DEPRESSED
PEACEFUL
LONELY
CONFUSED
HAPPY
SAD
DISAPPROVAL
EXCITED
SURPRISE
DISGUST
AWFUL
AMAZED
FEAR
ANGER
DISAPPOINTED
INSECURE
AGGRESSIVE
HUMILIATED
SCARED
HURT
MAD
THOUGHTS & INSIGHTS
QUALITY AND INTENSITY
FOCUS AND BREATHING
1 — 2 — 3 — 4 — 5 — 6 — 7 — 8 — 9 — 10
VISIONS AND EMOTIONS
REFLECTIONS
I am grateful for ...
I will accomplish ...
I need to work on ...

Notes

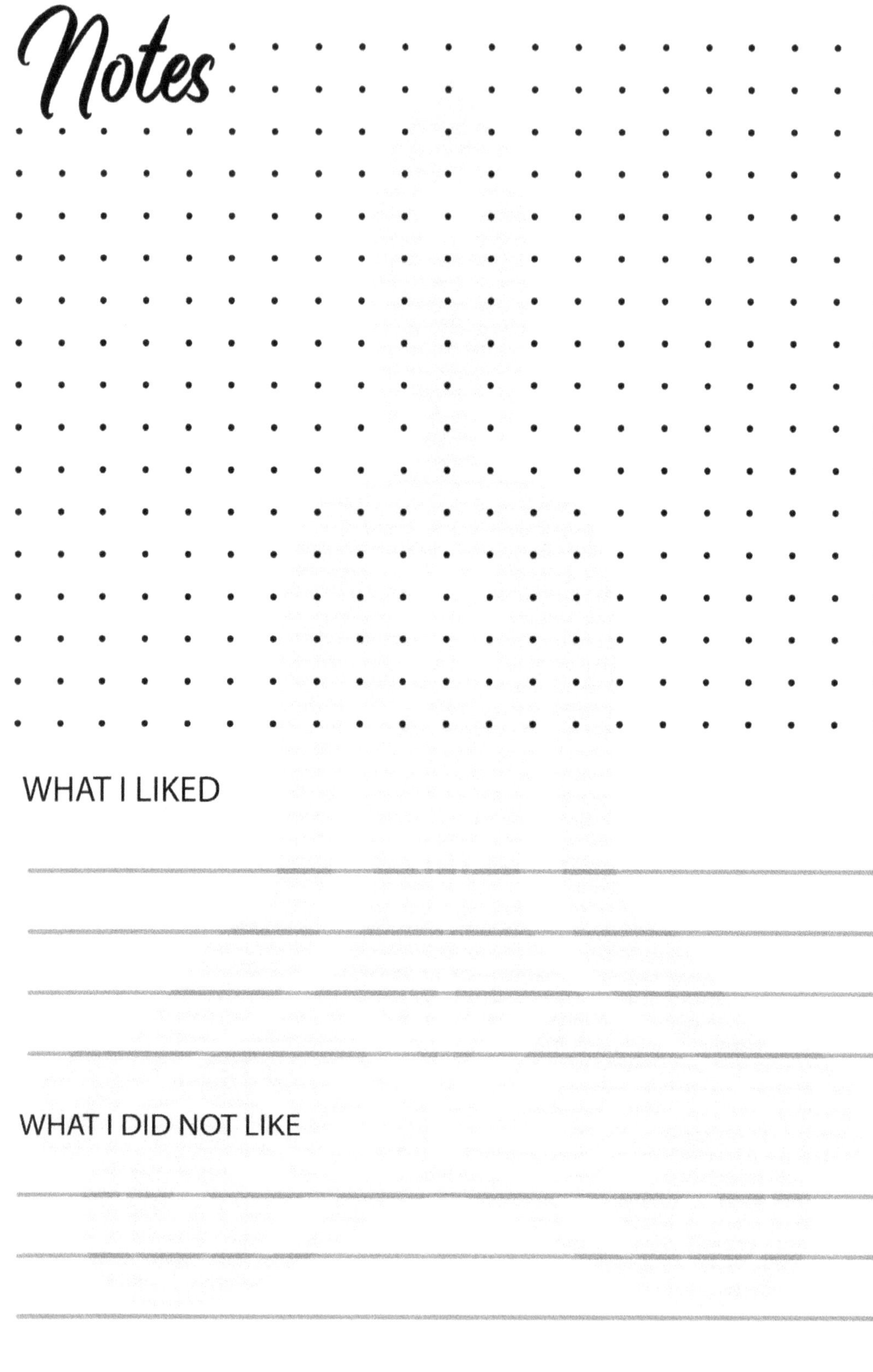

WHAT I LIKED

WHAT I DID NOT LIKE

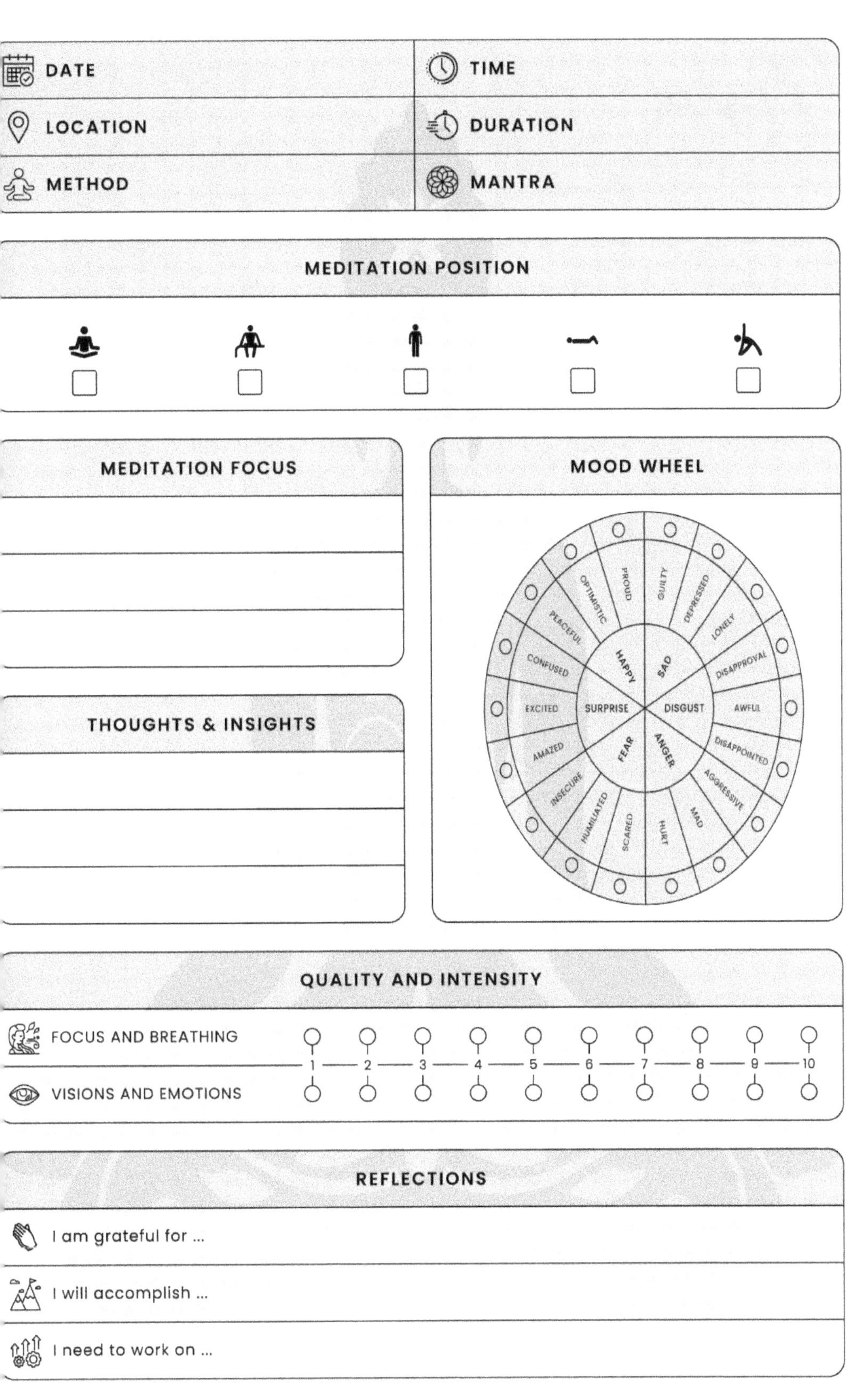

DATE
TIME
LOCATION
DURATION
METHOD
MANTRA
MEDITATION POSITION
MEDITATION FOCUS
MOOD WHEEL
OPTIMISTIC
PROUD
GUILTY
DEPRESSED
PEACEFUL
LONELY
CONFUSED
HAPPY
SAD
DISAPPROVAL
EXCITED
SURPRISE
DISGUST
AWFUL
AMAZED
FEAR
ANGER
DISAPPOINTED
INSECURE
AGGRESSIVE
HUMILIATED
SCARED
HURT
MAD
THOUGHTS & INSIGHTS
QUALITY AND INTENSITY
FOCUS AND BREATHING
1 — 2 — 3 — 4 — 5 — 6 — 7 — 8 — 9 — 10
VISIONS AND EMOTIONS
REFLECTIONS
I am grateful for ...
I will accomplish ...
I need to work on ...

Notes

WHAT I LIKED

WHAT I DID NOT LIKE

DATE

TIME

LOCATION

DURATION

METHOD

MANTRA

MEDITATION POSITION

MEDITATION FOCUS

MOOD WHEEL

THOUGHTS & INSIGHTS

QUALITY AND INTENSITY

FOCUS AND BREATHING

1 — 2 — 3 — 4 — 5 — 6 — 7 — 8 — 9 — 10

VISIONS AND EMOTIONS

REFLECTIONS

I am grateful for ...

I will accomplish ...

I need to work on ...

Notes

WHAT I LIKED

WHAT I DID NOT LIKE

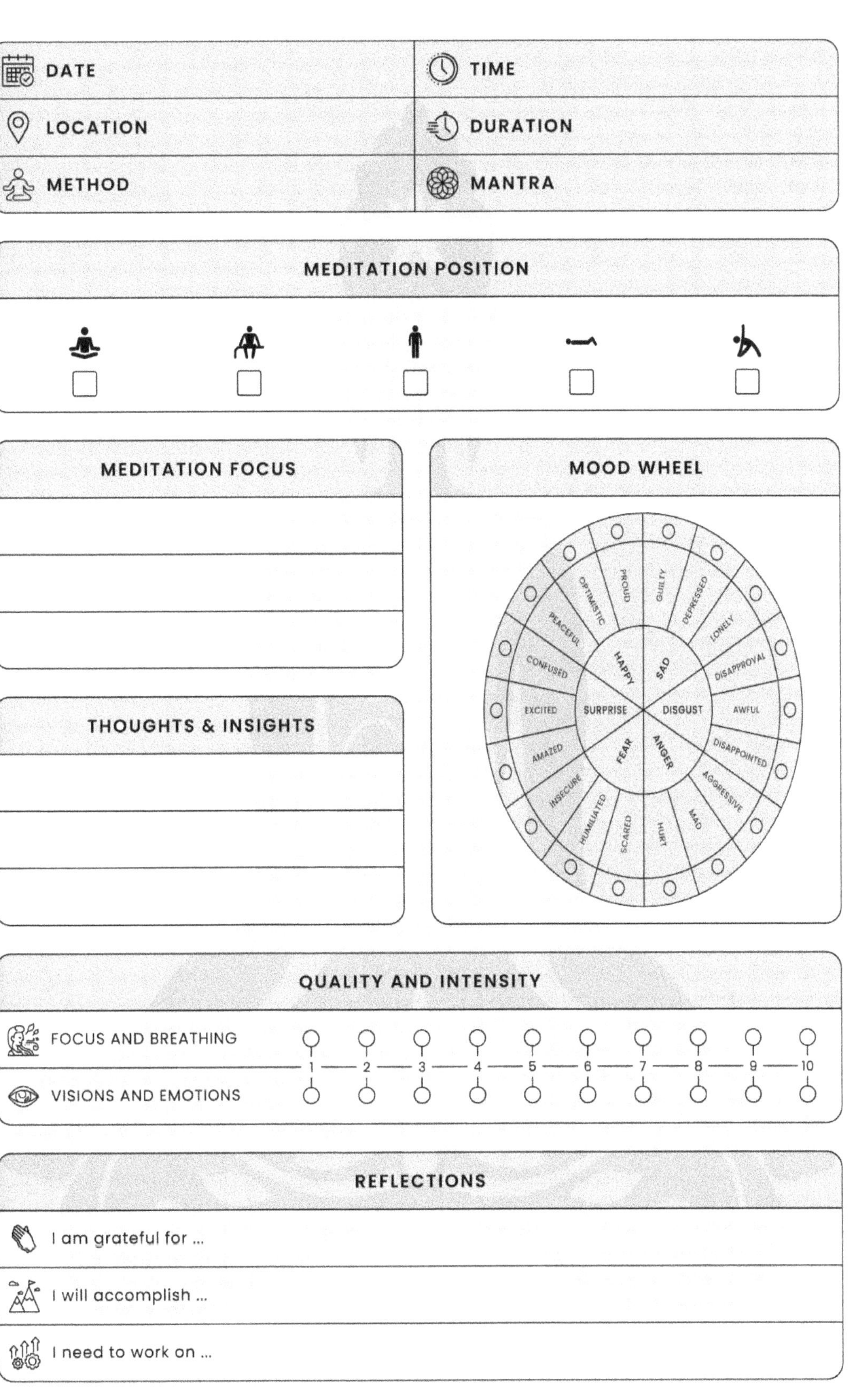

DATE
TIME
LOCATION
DURATION
METHOD
MANTRA

MEDITATION POSITION

MEDITATION FOCUS

MOOD WHEEL

OPTIMISTIC
PROUD
GUILTY
DEPRESSED
PEACEFUL
LONELY
CONFUSED
DISAPPROVAL
HAPPY
SAD
EXCITED
SURPRISE
DISGUST
AWFUL
AMAZED
FEAR
ANGER
DISAPPOINTED
INSECURE
AGGRESSIVE
HUMILIATED
SCARED
HURT
MAD

THOUGHTS & INSIGHTS

QUALITY AND INTENSITY

FOCUS AND BREATHING
1 — 2 — 3 — 4 — 5 — 6 — 7 — 8 — 9 — 10
VISIONS AND EMOTIONS

REFLECTIONS

I am grateful for ...

I will accomplish ...

I need to work on ...

Notes

WHAT I LIKED

WHAT I DID NOT LIKE

DATE		TIME	
LOCATION		DURATION	
METHOD		MANTRA	

MEDITATION POSITION

☐ ☐ ☐ ☐ ☐

MEDITATION FOCUS

THOUGHTS & INSIGHTS

MOOD WHEEL

QUALITY AND INTENSITY

FOCUS AND BREATHING

1 — 2 — 3 — 4 — 5 — 6 — 7 — 8 — 9 — 10

VISIONS AND EMOTIONS

REFLECTIONS

I am grateful for ...

I will accomplish ...

I need to work on ...

Notes

WHAT I LIKED

WHAT I DID NOT LIKE

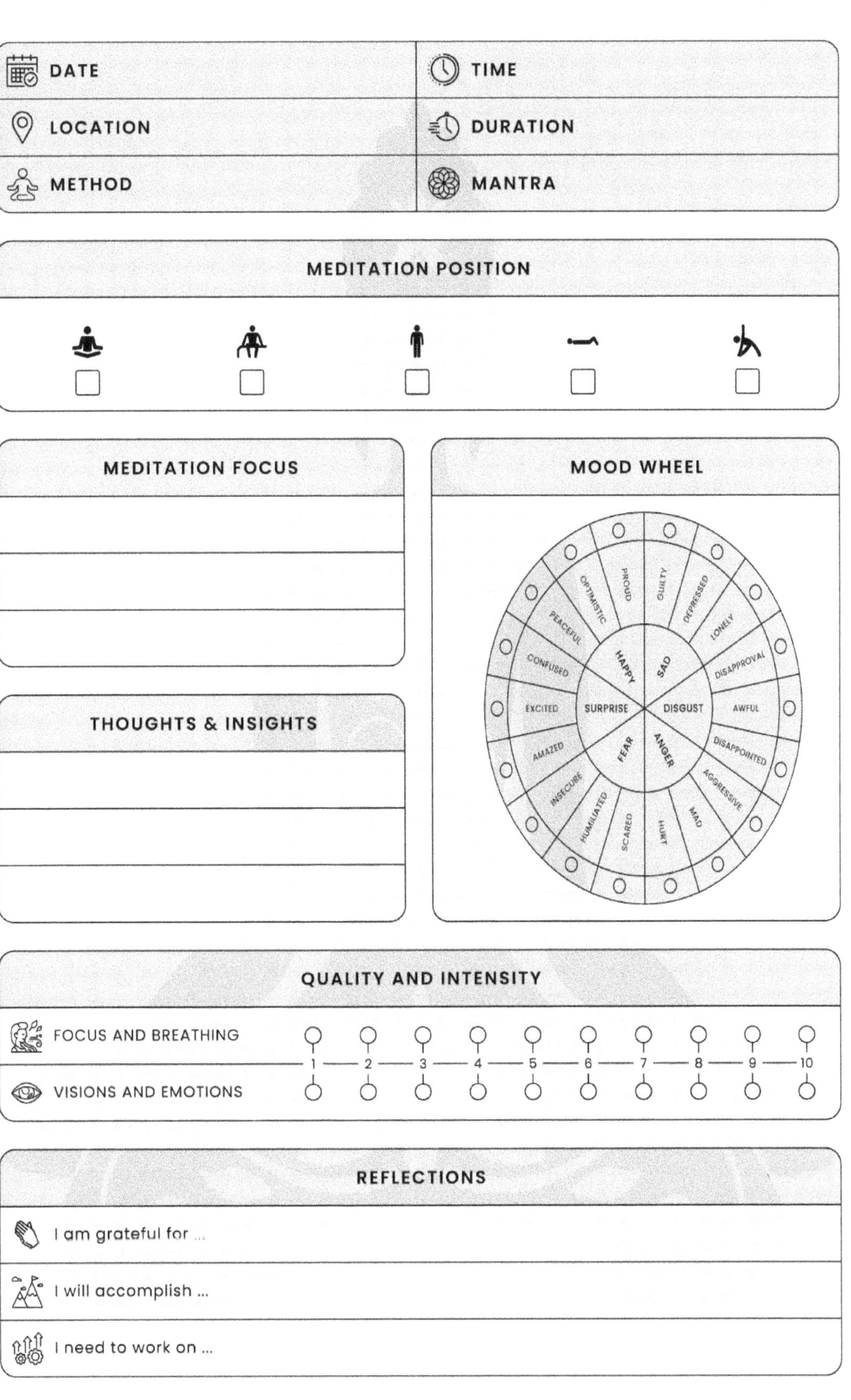

DATE
TIME
LOCATION
DURATION
METHOD
MANTRA

MEDITATION POSITION

MEDITATION FOCUS

MOOD WHEEL

OPTIMISTIC
PROUD
GUILTY
PEACEFUL
DEPRESSED
CONFUSED
LONELY
HAPPY
SAD
DISAPPROVAL
EXCITED
SURPRISE
DISGUST
AWFUL
AMAZED
FEAR
ANGER
DISAPPOINTED
INSECURE
AGGRESSIVE
HUMILIATED
SCARED
HURT
MAD

THOUGHTS & INSIGHTS

QUALITY AND INTENSITY

FOCUS AND BREATHING
1 — 2 — 3 — 4 — 5 — 6 — 7 — 8 — 9 — 10
VISIONS AND EMOTIONS

REFLECTIONS

I am grateful for ...

I will accomplish ...

I need to work on ...

Notes

WHAT I LIKED

WHAT I DID NOT LIKE

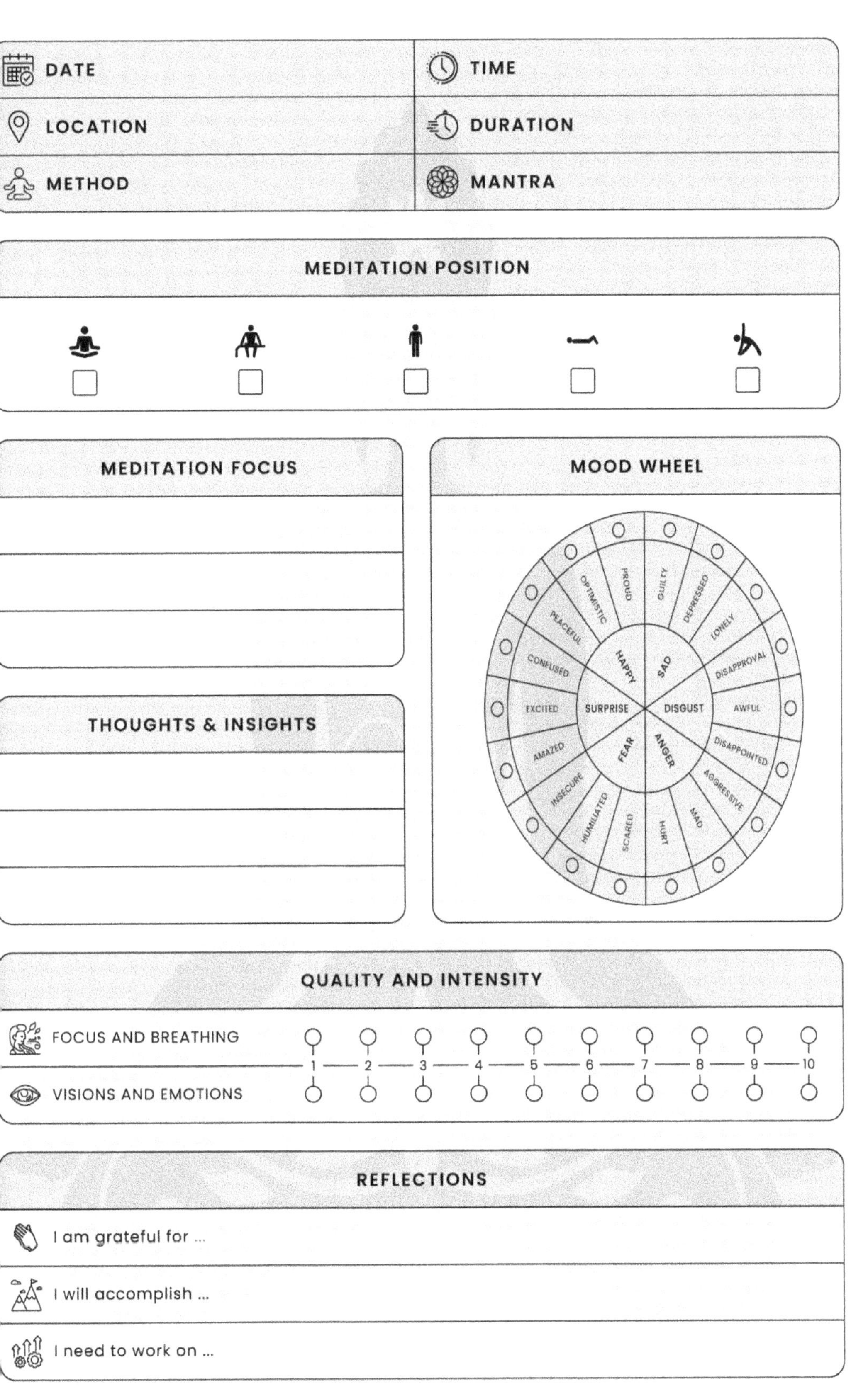

DATE
TIME
LOCATION
DURATION
METHOD
MANTRA

MEDITATION POSITION

MEDITATION FOCUS

MOOD WHEEL

OPTIMISTIC
PROUD
GUILTY
DEPRESSED
PEACEFUL
LONELY
CONFUSED
HAPPY
SAD
DISAPPROVAL
EXCITED
SURPRISE
DISGUST
AWFUL
AMAZED
FEAR
ANGER
DISAPPOINTED
INSECURE
AGGRESSIVE
HUMILIATED
SCARED
HURT
MAD

THOUGHTS & INSIGHTS

QUALITY AND INTENSITY

FOCUS AND BREATHING
1 — 2 — 3 — 4 — 5 — 6 — 7 — 8 — 9 — 10
VISIONS AND EMOTIONS

REFLECTIONS

I am grateful for ...

I will accomplish ...

I need to work on ...

Notes

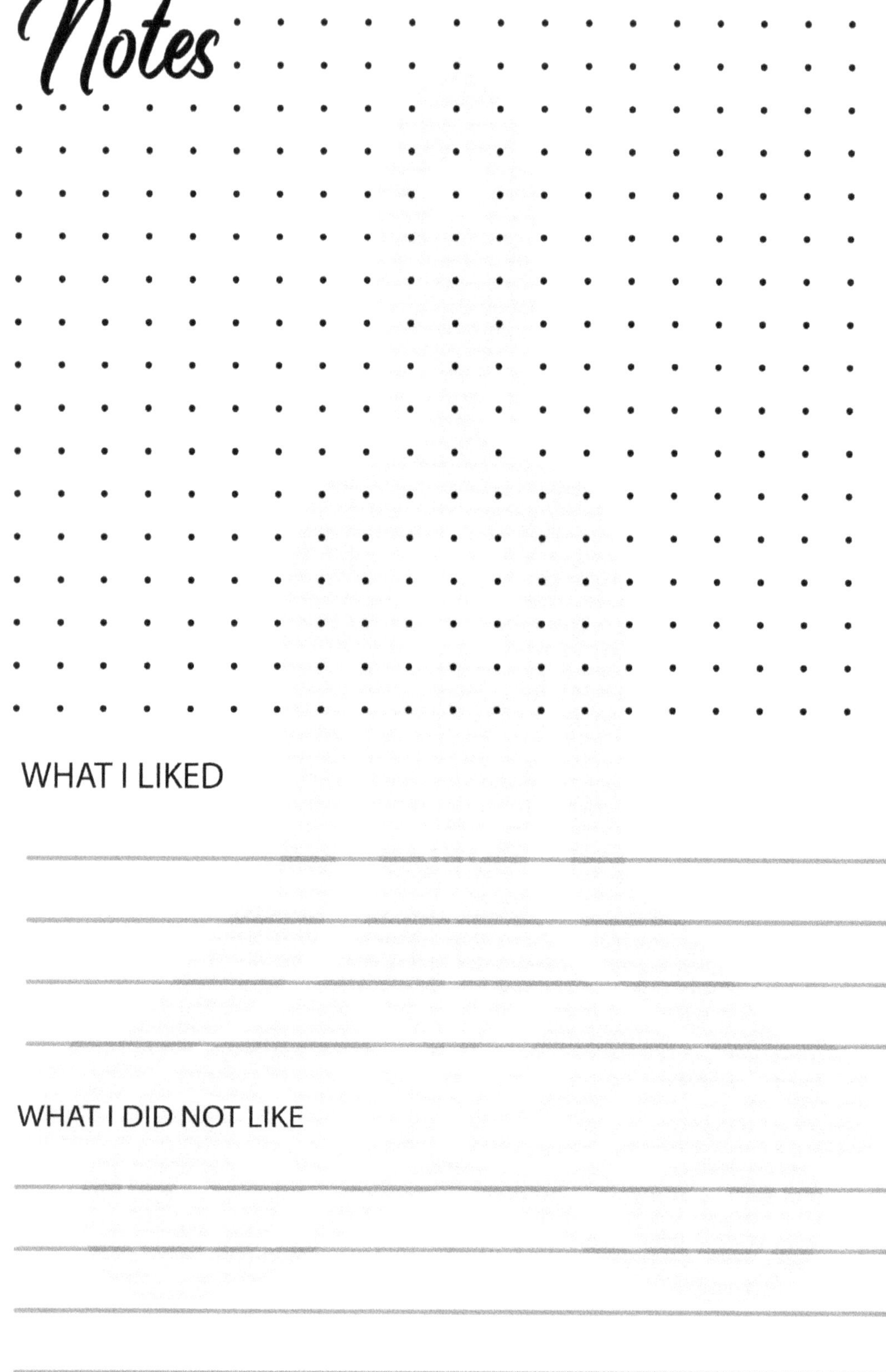

WHAT I LIKED

WHAT I DID NOT LIKE

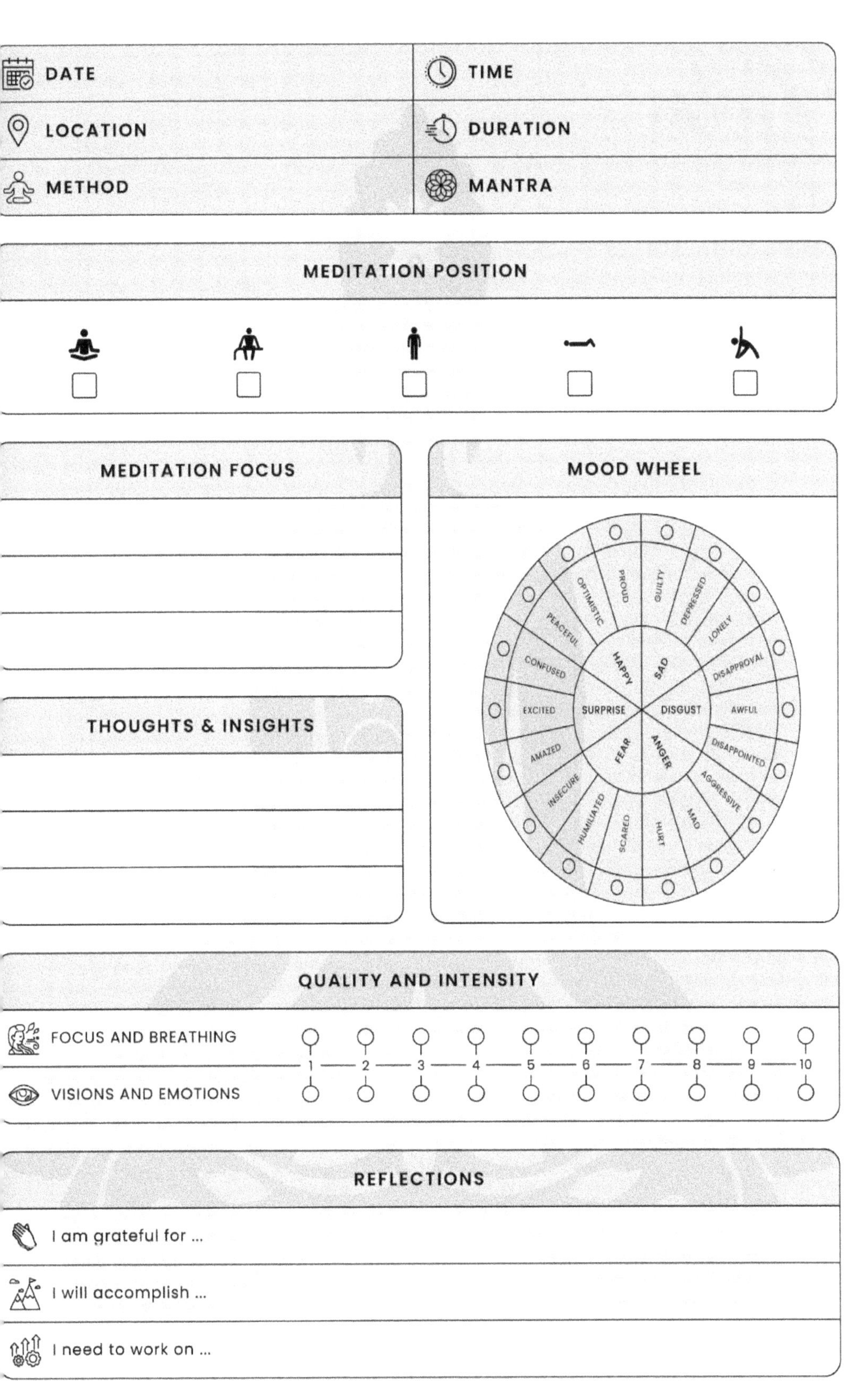

DATE
TIME
LOCATION
DURATION
METHOD
MANTRA

MEDITATION POSITION

MEDITATION FOCUS

MOOD WHEEL

OPTIMISTIC
PROUD
GUILTY
DEPRESSED
PEACEFUL
LONELY
CONFUSED
DISAPPROVAL
HAPPY
SAD
EXCITED
SURPRISE
DISGUST
AWFUL
AMAZED
FEAR
ANGER
DISAPPOINTED
INSECURE
AGGRESSIVE
HUMILIATED
SCARED
HURT
MAD

THOUGHTS & INSIGHTS

QUALITY AND INTENSITY

FOCUS AND BREATHING
1 — 2 — 3 — 4 — 5 — 6 — 7 — 8 — 9 — 10
VISIONS AND EMOTIONS

REFLECTIONS

I am grateful for ...

I will accomplish ...

I need to work on ...

Notes

WHAT I LIKED

WHAT I DID NOT LIKE

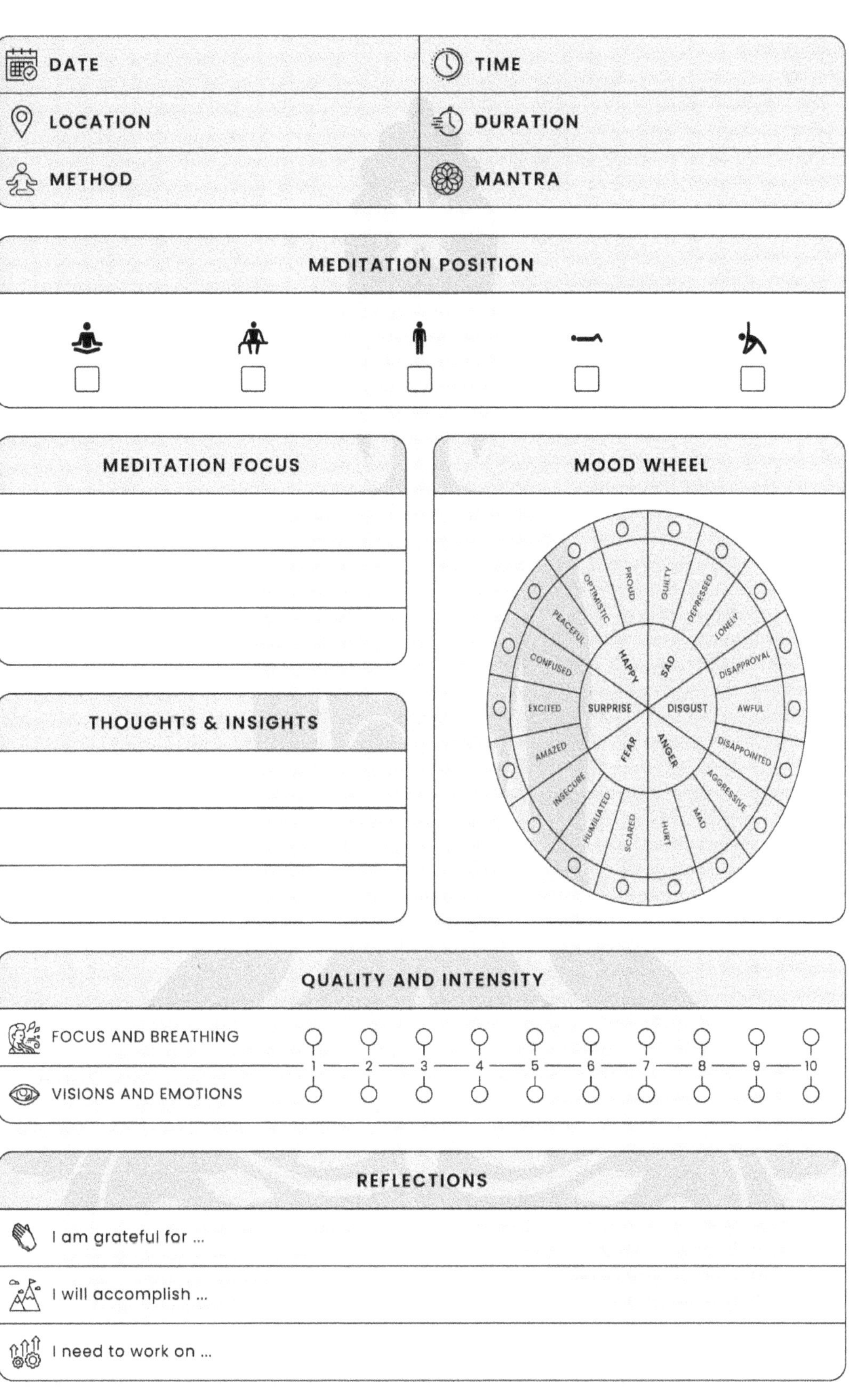

DATE
TIME
LOCATION
DURATION
METHOD
MANTRA

MEDITATION POSITION

MEDITATION FOCUS

MOOD WHEEL

OPTIMISTIC
PROUD
GUILTY
DEPRESSED
PEACEFUL
LONELY
CONFUSED
HAPPY
SAD
DISAPPROVAL
EXCITED
SURPRISE
DISGUST
AWFUL
AMAZED
FEAR
ANGER
DISAPPOINTED
INSECURE
AGGRESSIVE
HUMILIATED
SCARED
HURT
MAD

THOUGHTS & INSIGHTS

QUALITY AND INTENSITY

FOCUS AND BREATHING
1 — 2 — 3 — 4 — 5 — 6 — 7 — 8 — 9 — 10
VISIONS AND EMOTIONS

REFLECTIONS

I am grateful for ...

I will accomplish ...

I need to work on ...

Notes

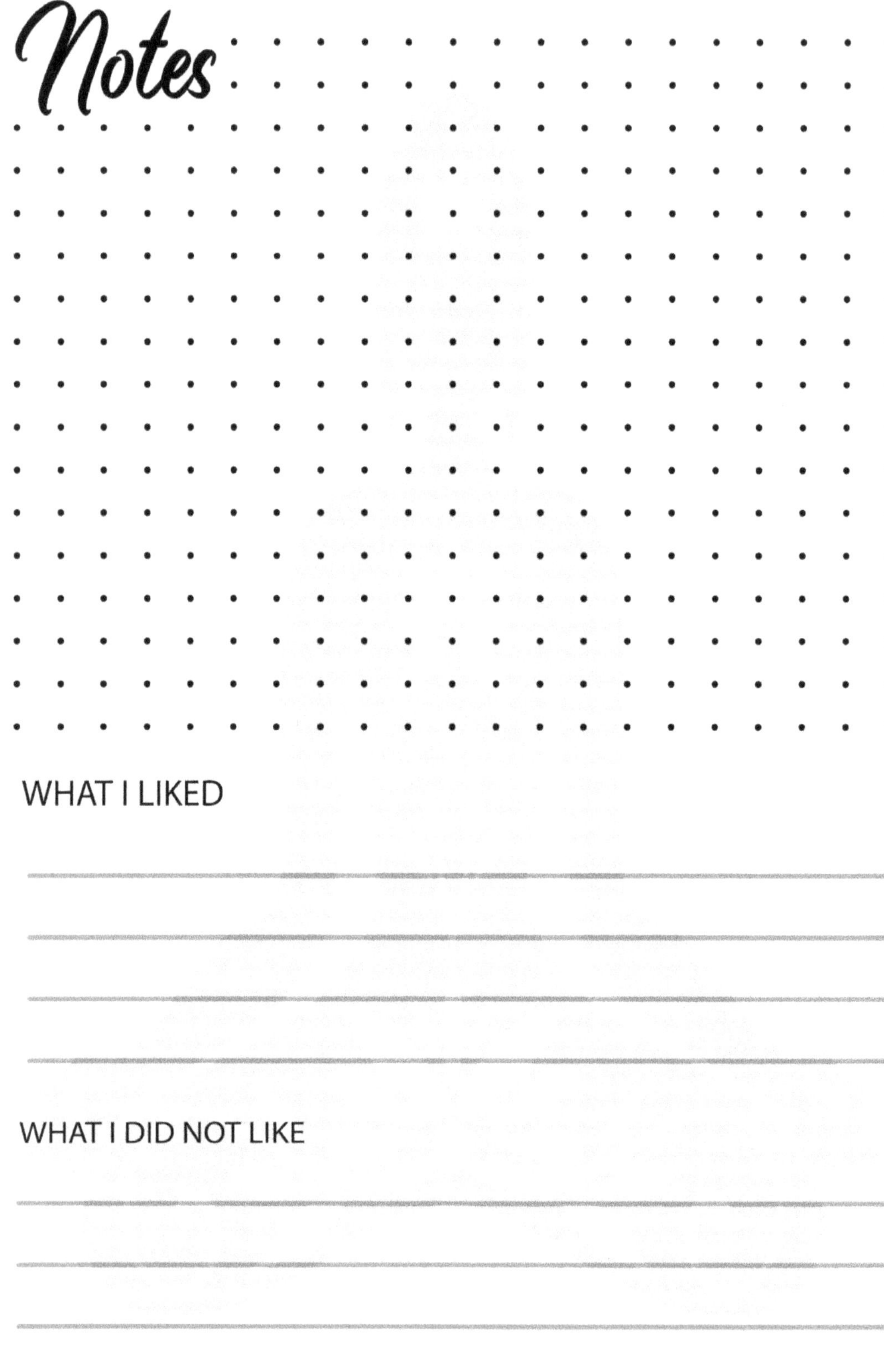

WHAT I LIKED

WHAT I DID NOT LIKE

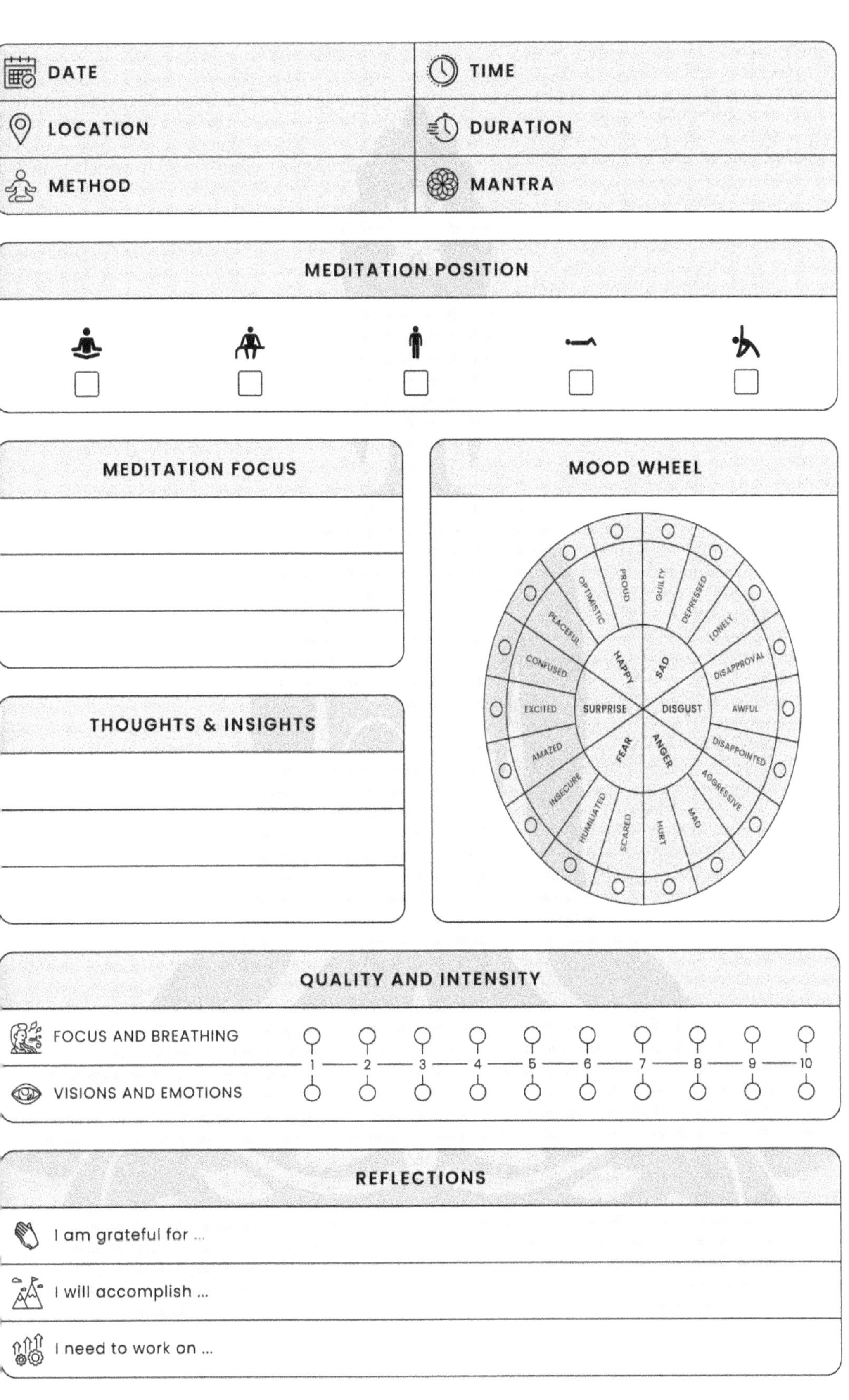

 📅 **DATE**	🕐 **TIME**
📍 **LOCATION**	⏱️ **DURATION**
🧘 **METHOD**	✿ **MANTRA**

MEDITATION POSITION

☐ ☐ ☐ ☐ ☐

MEDITATION FOCUS

THOUGHTS & INSIGHTS

MOOD WHEEL

QUALITY AND INTENSITY

FOCUS AND BREATHING

1 — 2 — 3 — 4 — 5 — 6 — 7 — 8 — 9 — 10

VISIONS AND EMOTIONS

REFLECTIONS

🖐️ I am grateful for ...

⛰️ I will accomplish ...

⚙️ I need to work on ...

Notes

WHAT I LIKED

WHAT I DID NOT LIKE

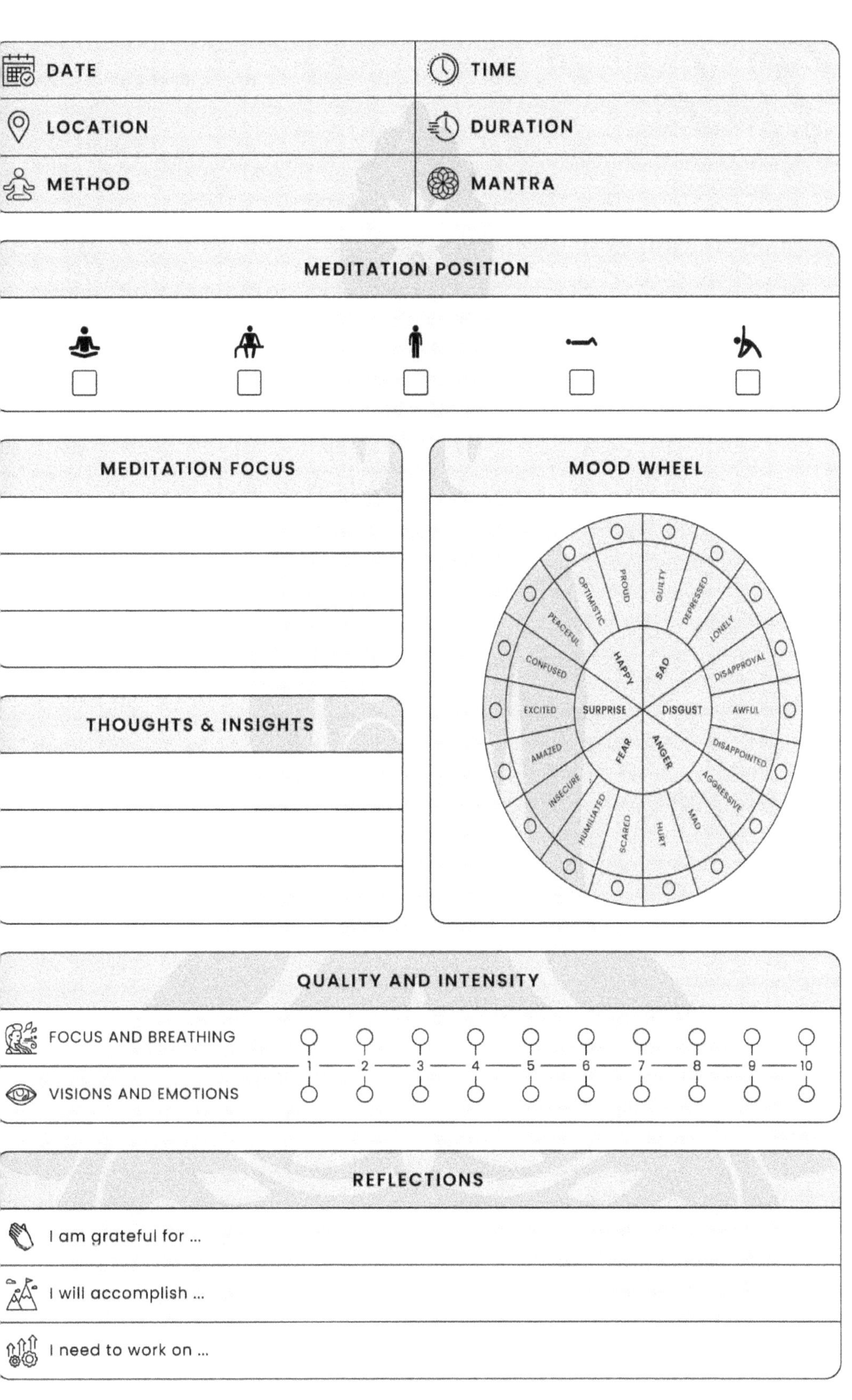

DATE
TIME
LOCATION
DURATION
METHOD
MANTRA
MEDITATION POSITION
MEDITATION FOCUS
MOOD WHEEL
OPTIMISTIC
PROUD
GUILTY
DEPRESSED
PEACEFUL
LONELY
CONFUSED
HAPPY
SAD
DISAPPROVAL
EXCITED
SURPRISE
DISGUST
AWFUL
AMAZED
FEAR
ANGER
DISAPPOINTED
INSECURE
AGGRESSIVE
HUMILIATED
SCARED
HURT
MAD
THOUGHTS & INSIGHTS
QUALITY AND INTENSITY
FOCUS AND BREATHING
1 2 3 4 5 6 7 8 9 10
VISIONS AND EMOTIONS
REFLECTIONS
I am grateful for ...
I will accomplish ...
I need to work on ...

Notes

WHAT I LIKED

WHAT I DID NOT LIKE

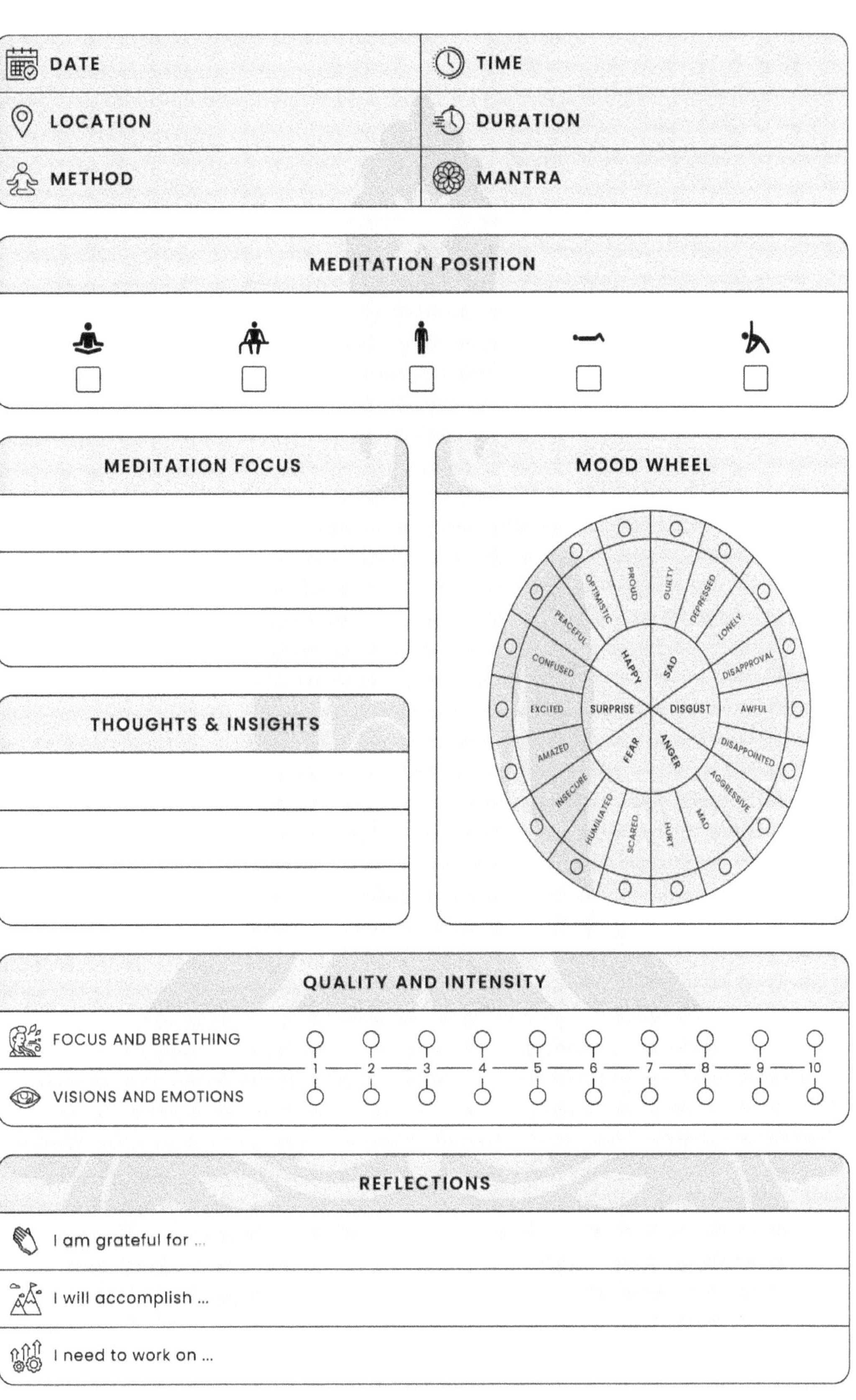
DATE
TIME
LOCATION
DURATION
METHOD
MANTRA

MEDITATION POSITION

MEDITATION FOCUS

MOOD WHEEL

OPTIMISTIC
PROUD
GUILTY
DEPRESSED
PEACEFUL
LONELY
CONFUSED
HAPPY
SAD
DISAPPROVAL
EXCITED
SURPRISE
DISGUST
AWFUL
AMAZED
FEAR
ANGER
DISAPPOINTED
INSECURE
AGGRESSIVE
HUMILIATED
SCARED
HURT
MAD

THOUGHTS & INSIGHTS

QUALITY AND INTENSITY

FOCUS AND BREATHING
1 — 2 — 3 — 4 — 5 — 6 — 7 — 8 — 9 — 10
VISIONS AND EMOTIONS

REFLECTIONS

I am grateful for ...

I will accomplish ...

I need to work on ...

Notes

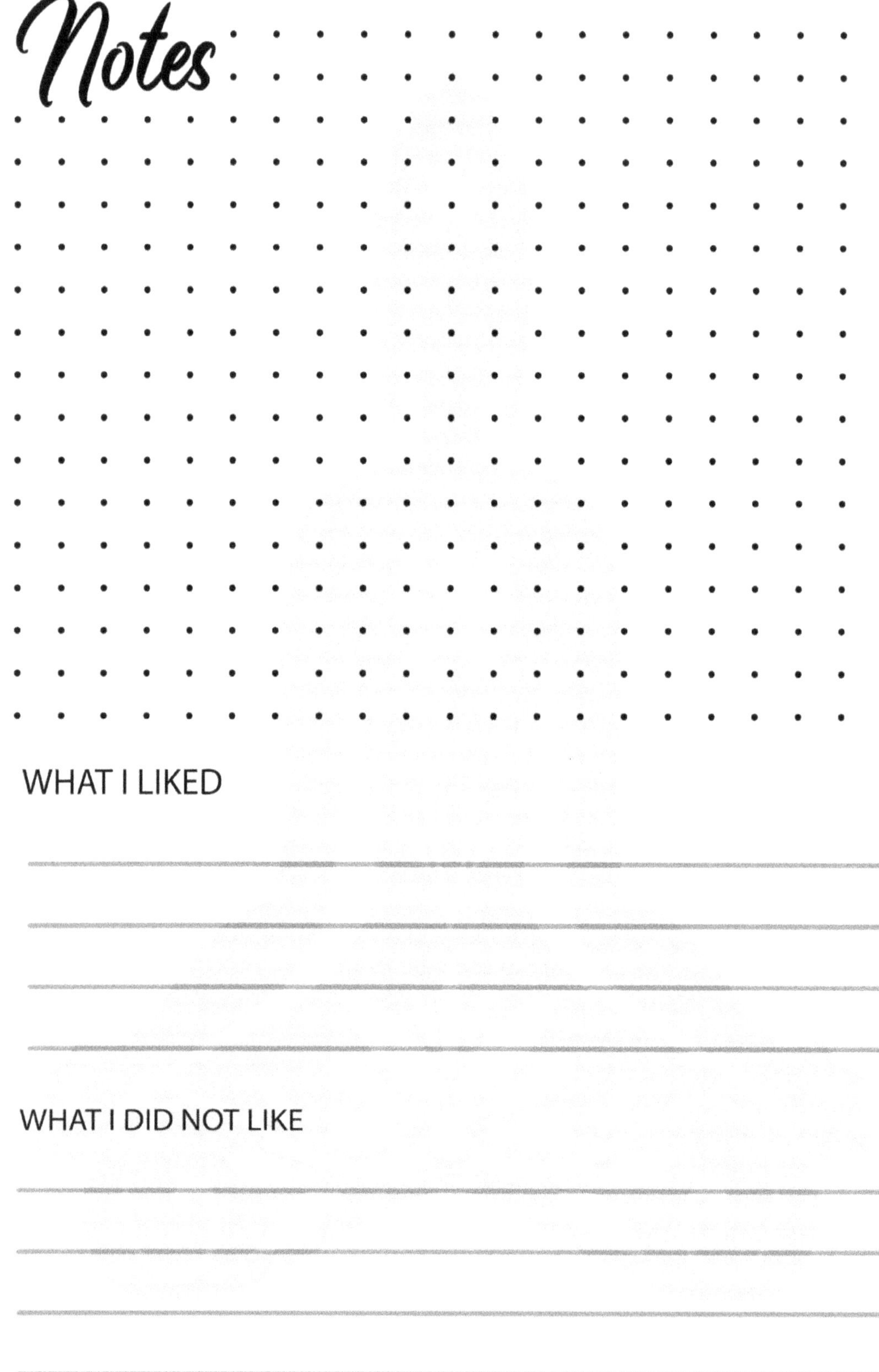

WHAT I LIKED

WHAT I DID NOT LIKE

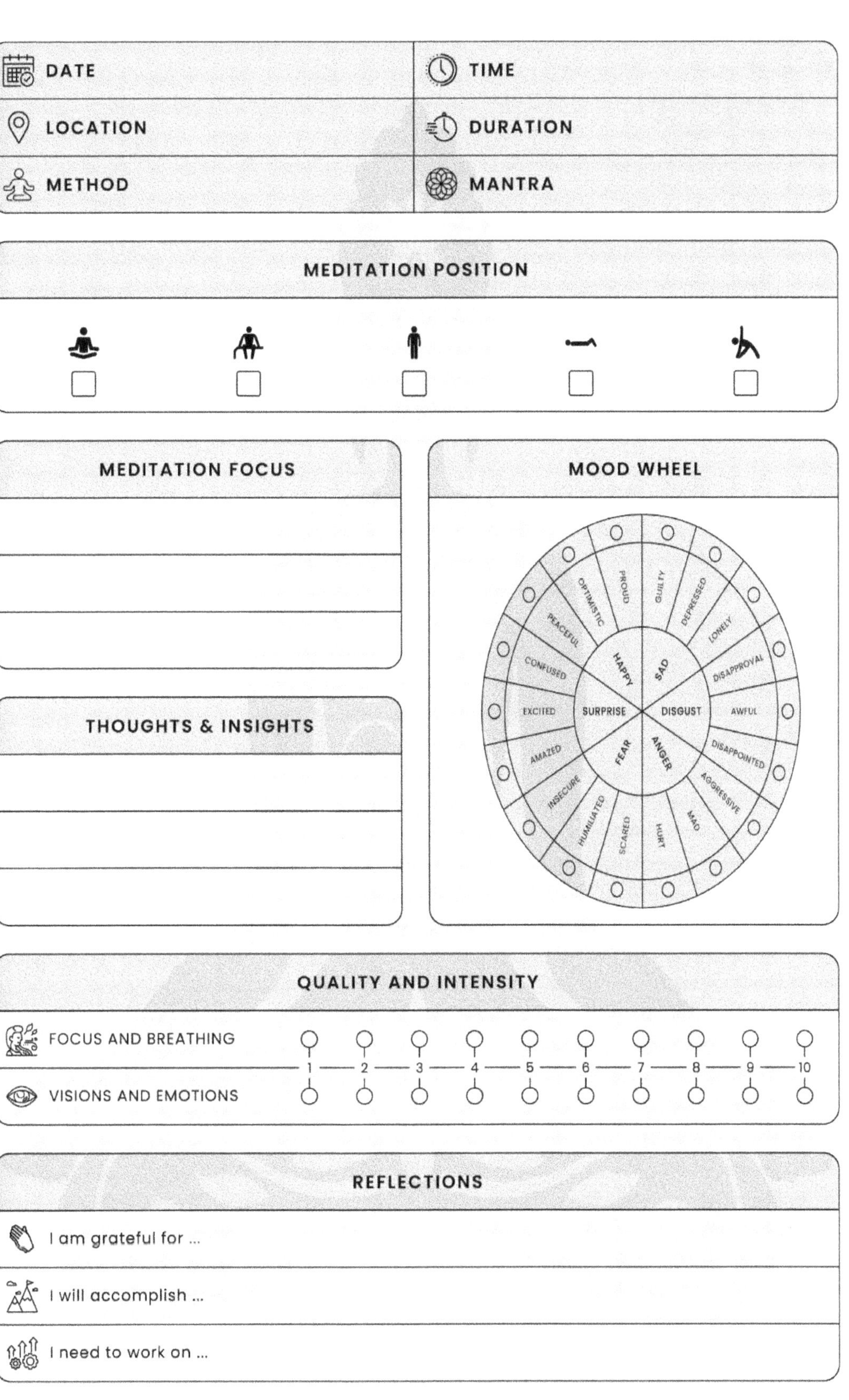

DATE
TIME
LOCATION
DURATION
METHOD
MANTRA

MEDITATION POSITION

MEDITATION FOCUS

MOOD WHEEL

OPTIMISTIC
PROUD
GUILTY
DEPRESSED
PEACEFUL
LONELY
CONFUSED
DISAPPROVAL
HAPPY
SAD
EXCITED
SURPRISE
DISGUST
AWFUL
AMAZED
FEAR
ANGER
DISAPPOINTED
INSECURE
AGGRESSIVE
HUMILIATED
SCARED
HURT
MAD

THOUGHTS & INSIGHTS

QUALITY AND INTENSITY

FOCUS AND BREATHING
1 — 2 — 3 — 4 — 5 — 6 — 7 — 8 — 9 — 10
VISIONS AND EMOTIONS

REFLECTIONS

I am grateful for ...

I will accomplish ...

I need to work on ...

Notes

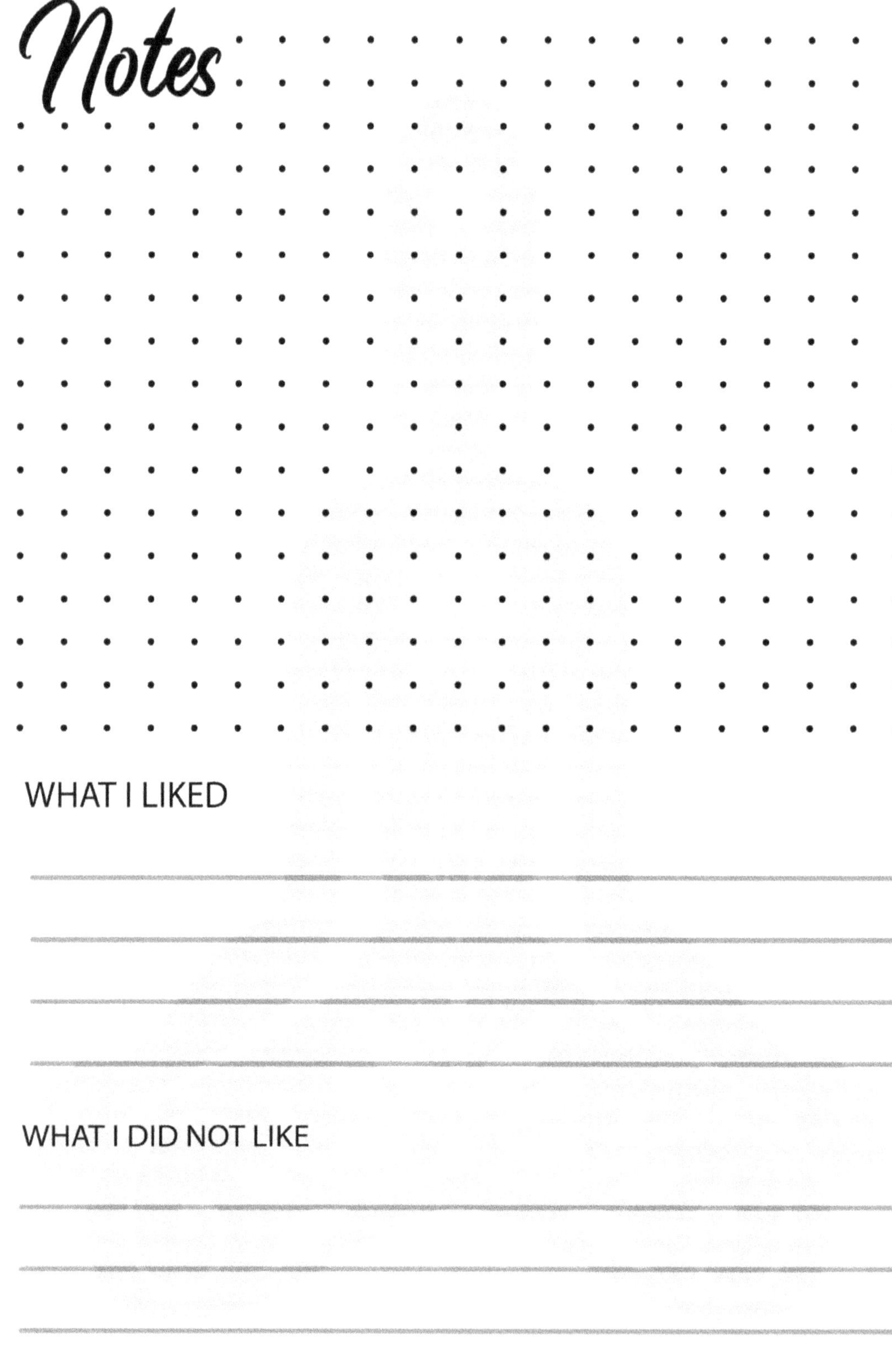

WHAT I LIKED

WHAT I DID NOT LIKE

MEDITATION POSITION

MEDITATION FOCUS

MOOD WHEEL

THOUGHTS & INSIGHTS

QUALITY AND INTENSITY

FOCUS AND BREATHING

1 — 2 — 3 — 4 — 5 — 6 — 7 — 8 — 9 — 10

VISIONS AND EMOTIONS

REFLECTIONS

I am grateful for ...

I will accomplish ...

I need to work on ...

Notes

WHAT I LIKED

WHAT I DID NOT LIKE

MEDITATION POSITION

MEDITATION FOCUS

MOOD WHEEL

THOUGHTS & INSIGHTS

QUALITY AND INTENSITY

FOCUS AND BREATHING

1 — 2 — 3 — 4 — 5 — 6 — 7 — 8 — 9 — 10

VISIONS AND EMOTIONS

REFLECTIONS

I am grateful for ...

I will accomplish ...

I need to work on ...

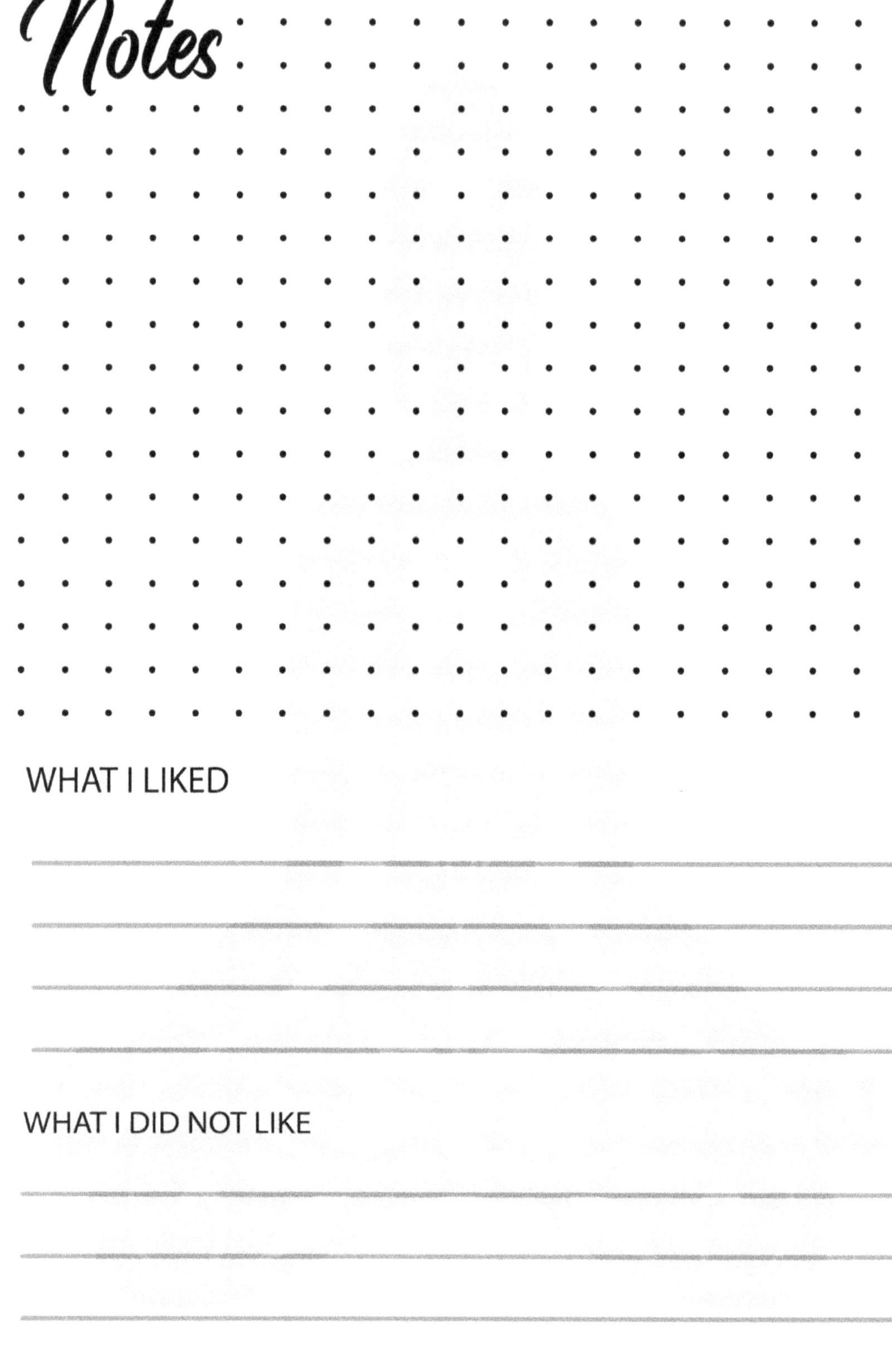

Notes

WHAT I LIKED

WHAT I DID NOT LIKE

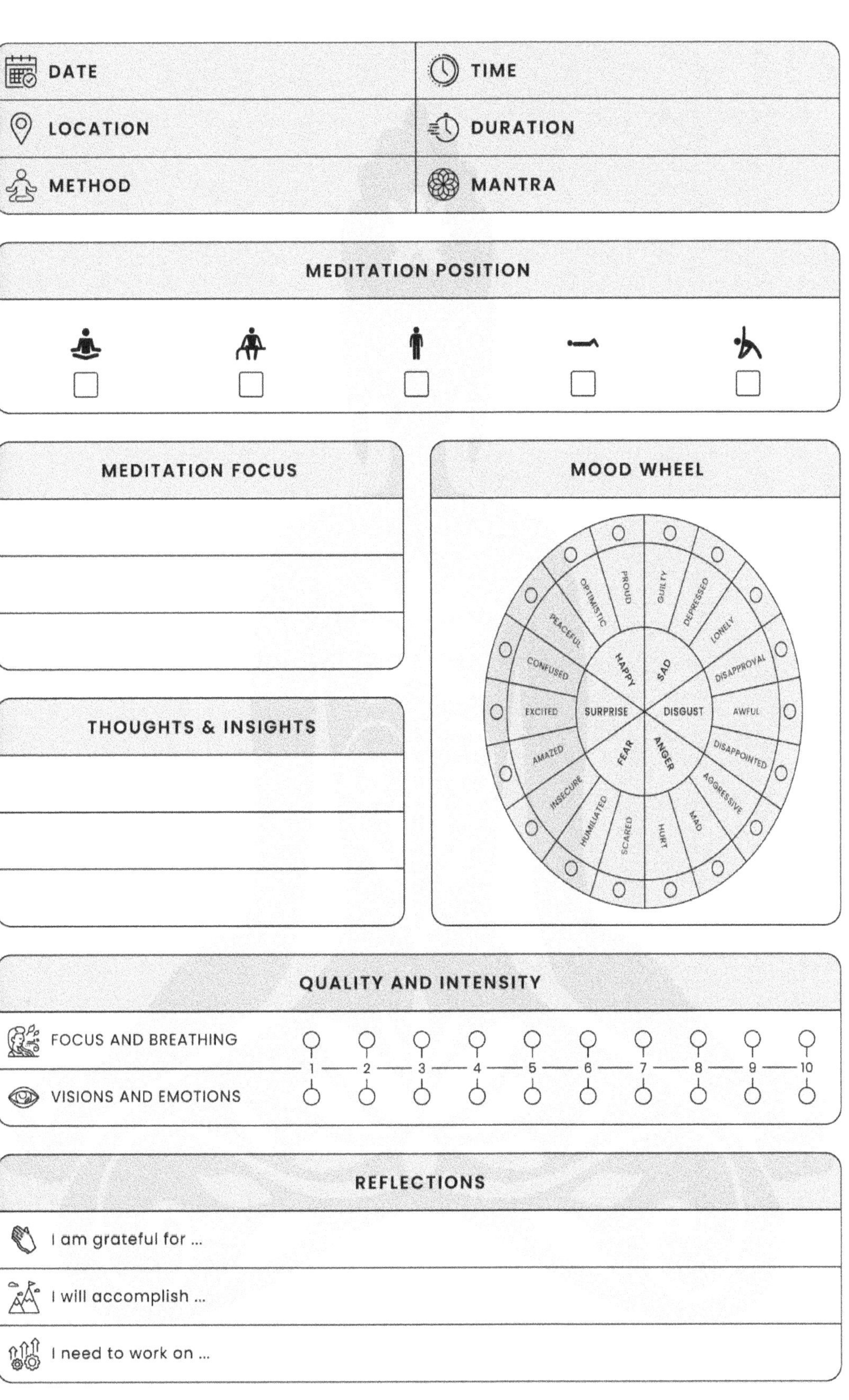

DATE
TIME
LOCATION
DURATION
METHOD
MANTRA

MEDITATION POSITION

MEDITATION FOCUS

THOUGHTS & INSIGHTS

MOOD WHEEL

OPTIMISTIC
PROUD
GUILTY
DEPRESSED
PEACEFUL
LONELY
CONFUSED
DISAPPROVAL
HAPPY
SAD
EXCITED
SURPRISE
DISGUST
AWFUL
AMAZED
FEAR
ANGER
DISAPPOINTED
INSECURE
AGGRESSIVE
HUMILIATED
SCARED
HURT
MAD

QUALITY AND INTENSITY

FOCUS AND BREATHING
1 — 2 — 3 — 4 — 5 — 6 — 7 — 8 — 9 — 10
VISIONS AND EMOTIONS

REFLECTIONS

I am grateful for ...

I will accomplish ...

I need to work on ...

Notes

WHAT I LIKED

WHAT I DID NOT LIKE

<table>
<tr><td>📅 DATE</td><td>🕐 TIME</td></tr>
<tr><td>📍 LOCATION</td><td>⏱ DURATION</td></tr>
<tr><td>🧘 METHOD</td><td>✾ MANTRA</td></tr>
</table>

MEDITATION POSITION

☐ ☐ ☐ ☐ ☐

MEDITATION FOCUS

MOOD WHEEL

THOUGHTS & INSIGHTS

QUALITY AND INTENSITY

FOCUS AND BREATHING

1 — 2 — 3 — 4 — 5 — 6 — 7 — 8 — 9 — 10

VISIONS AND EMOTIONS

REFLECTIONS

I am grateful for ...

I will accomplish ...

I need to work on ...

Notes

WHAT I LIKED

WHAT I DID NOT LIKE

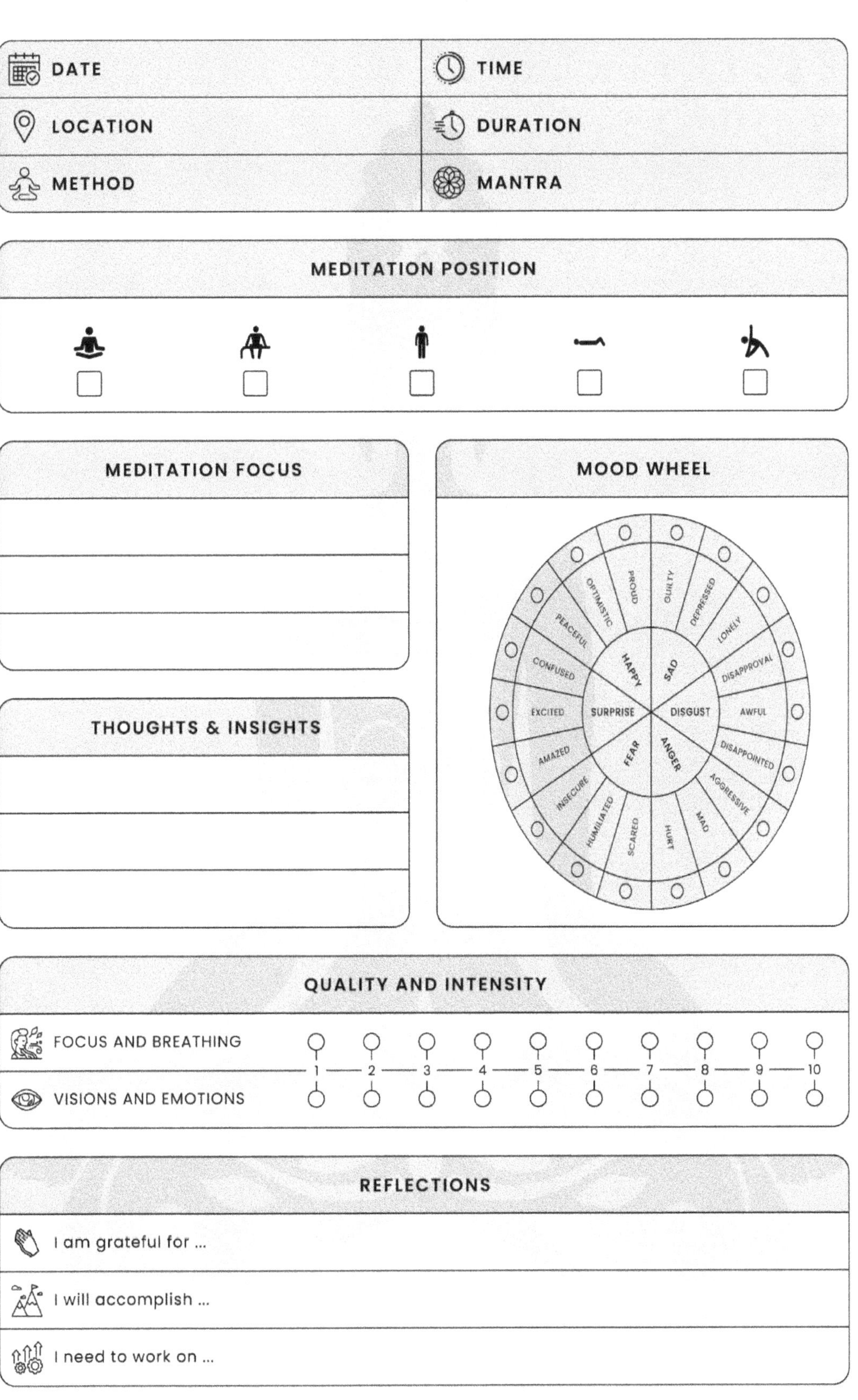

DATE	TIME
LOCATION	DURATION
METHOD	MANTRA

MEDITATION POSITION

☐ ☐ ☐ ☐ ☐

MEDITATION FOCUS

THOUGHTS & INSIGHTS

MOOD WHEEL

QUALITY AND INTENSITY

FOCUS AND BREATHING

1 — 2 — 3 — 4 — 5 — 6 — 7 — 8 — 9 — 10

VISIONS AND EMOTIONS

REFLECTIONS

I am grateful for ...

I will accomplish ...

I need to work on ...

Notes

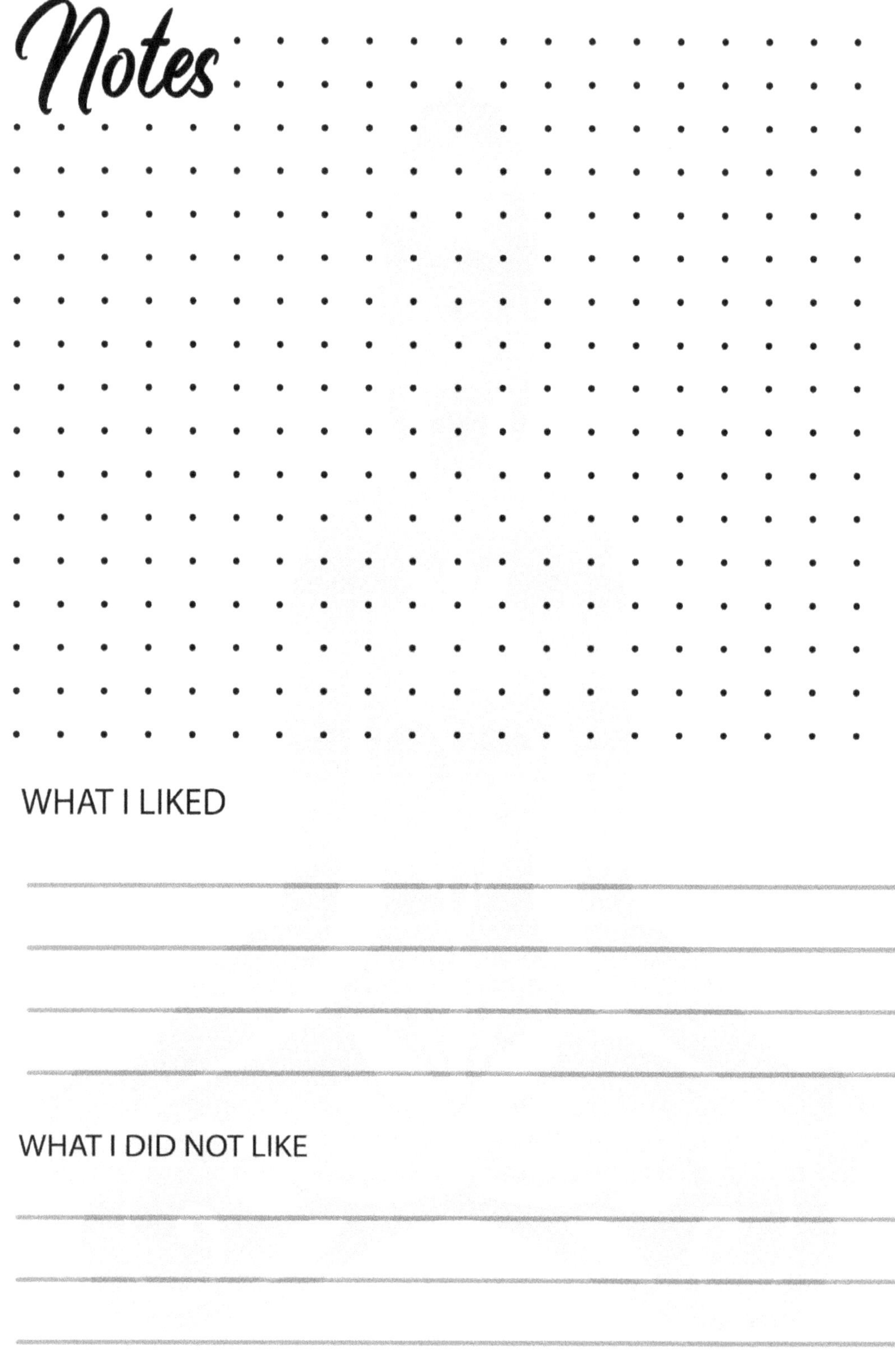

WHAT I LIKED

WHAT I DID NOT LIKE

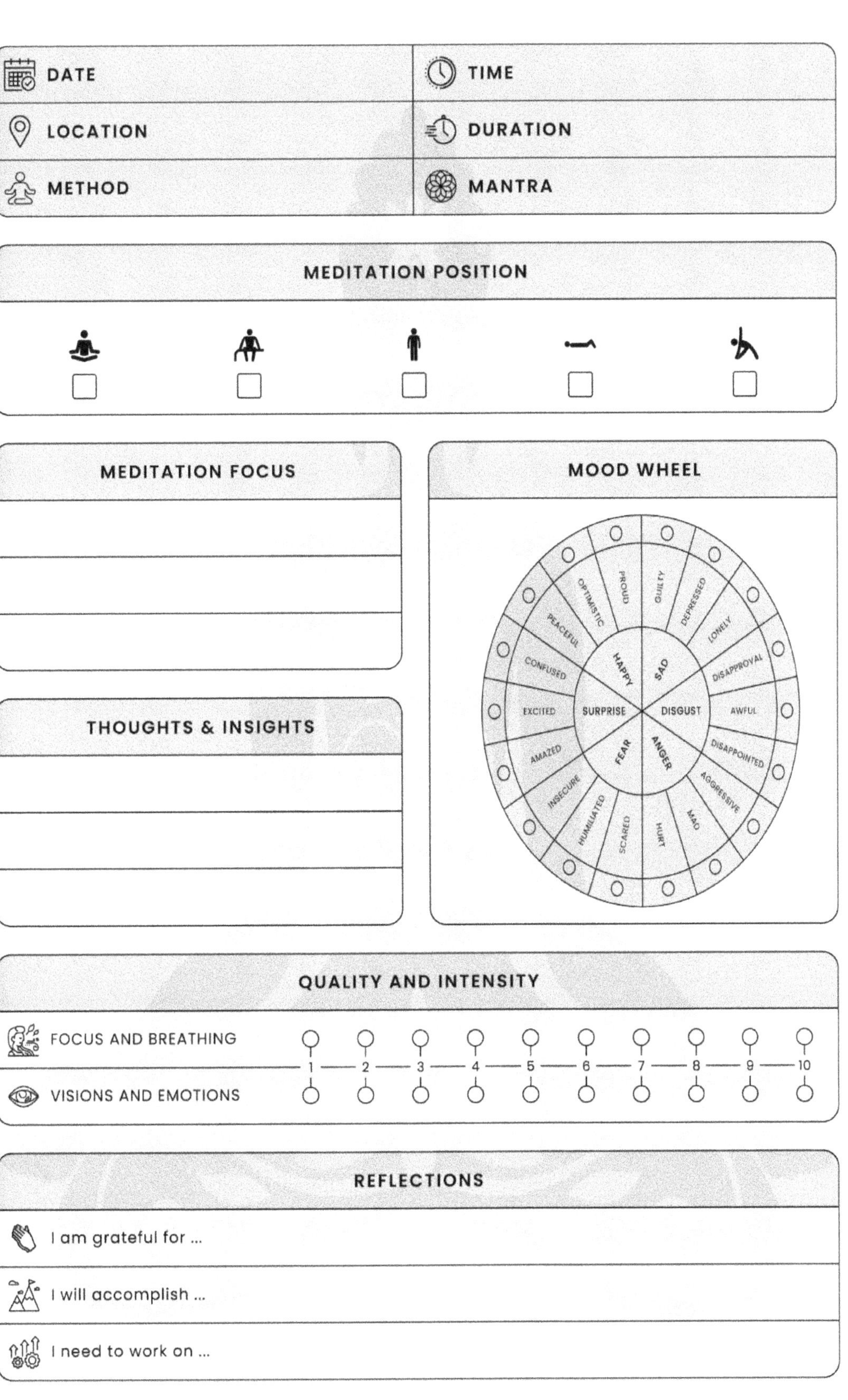

DATE
TIME
LOCATION
DURATION
METHOD
MANTRA

MEDITATION POSITION

MEDITATION FOCUS

MOOD WHEEL

OPTIMISTIC
PROUD
GUILTY
DEPRESSED
PEACEFUL
LONELY
CONFUSED
DISAPPROVAL
HAPPY
SAD
EXCITED
SURPRISE
DISGUST
AWFUL
AMAZED
FEAR
ANGER
DISAPPOINTED
INSECURE
AGGRESSIVE
HUMILIATED
SCARED
HURT
MAD

THOUGHTS & INSIGHTS

QUALITY AND INTENSITY

FOCUS AND BREATHING
1 — 2 — 3 — 4 — 5 — 6 — 7 — 8 — 9 — 10
VISIONS AND EMOTIONS

REFLECTIONS

I am grateful for ...

I will accomplish ...

I need to work on ...

Notes

WHAT I LIKED

WHAT I DID NOT LIKE

MEDITATION POSITION

MEDITATION FOCUS

THOUGHTS & INSIGHTS

MOOD WHEEL

QUALITY AND INTENSITY

FOCUS AND BREATHING

1 — 2 — 3 — 4 — 5 — 6 — 7 — 8 — 9 — 10

VISIONS AND EMOTIONS

REFLECTIONS

I am grateful for ...

I will accomplish ...

I need to work on ...

Notes

WHAT I LIKED

WHAT I DID NOT LIKE

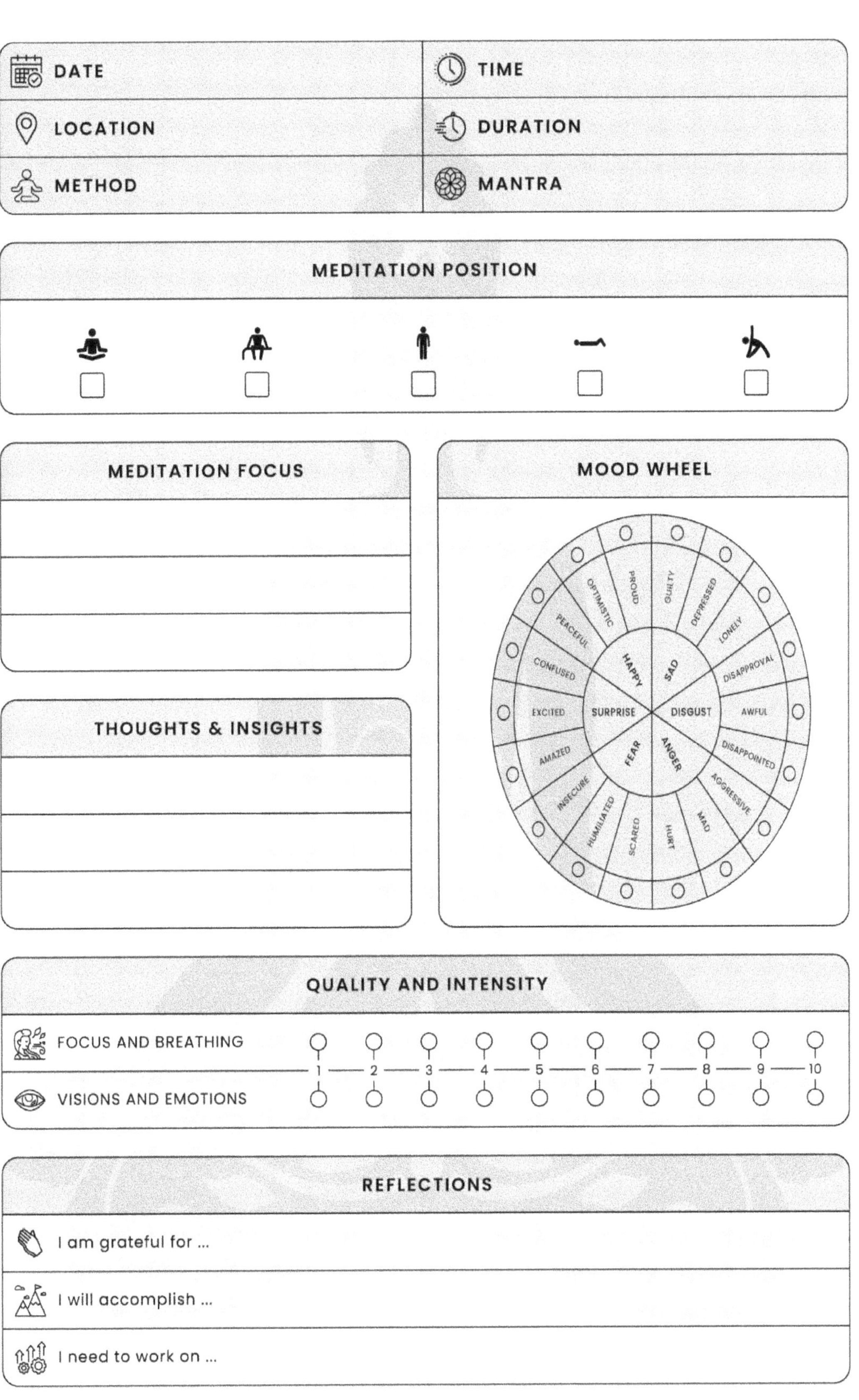
DATE
TIME
LOCATION
DURATION
METHOD
MANTRA

MEDITATION POSITION

MEDITATION FOCUS

MOOD WHEEL

OPTIMISTIC
PROUD
GUILTY
DEPRESSED
PEACEFUL
LONELY
CONFUSED
HAPPY
SAD
DISAPPROVAL
EXCITED
SURPRISE
DISGUST
AWFUL
AMAZED
FEAR
ANGER
DISAPPOINTED
INSECURE
AGGRESSIVE
HUMILIATED
SCARED
HURT
MAD

THOUGHTS & INSIGHTS

QUALITY AND INTENSITY

FOCUS AND BREATHING
1 — 2 — 3 — 4 — 5 — 6 — 7 — 8 — 9 — 10
VISIONS AND EMOTIONS

REFLECTIONS

I am grateful for ...

I will accomplish ...

I need to work on ...

Notes

WHAT I LIKED

WHAT I DID NOT LIKE

DATE	TIME
LOCATION	DURATION
METHOD	MANTRA

MEDITATION POSITION

MEDITATION FOCUS

THOUGHTS & INSIGHTS

MOOD WHEEL

QUALITY AND INTENSITY

FOCUS AND BREATHING

1 — 2 — 3 — 4 — 5 — 6 — 7 — 8 — 9 — 10

VISIONS AND EMOTIONS

REFLECTIONS

I am grateful for ...

I will accomplish ...

I need to work on ...

Notes

WHAT I LIKED

WHAT I DID NOT LIKE

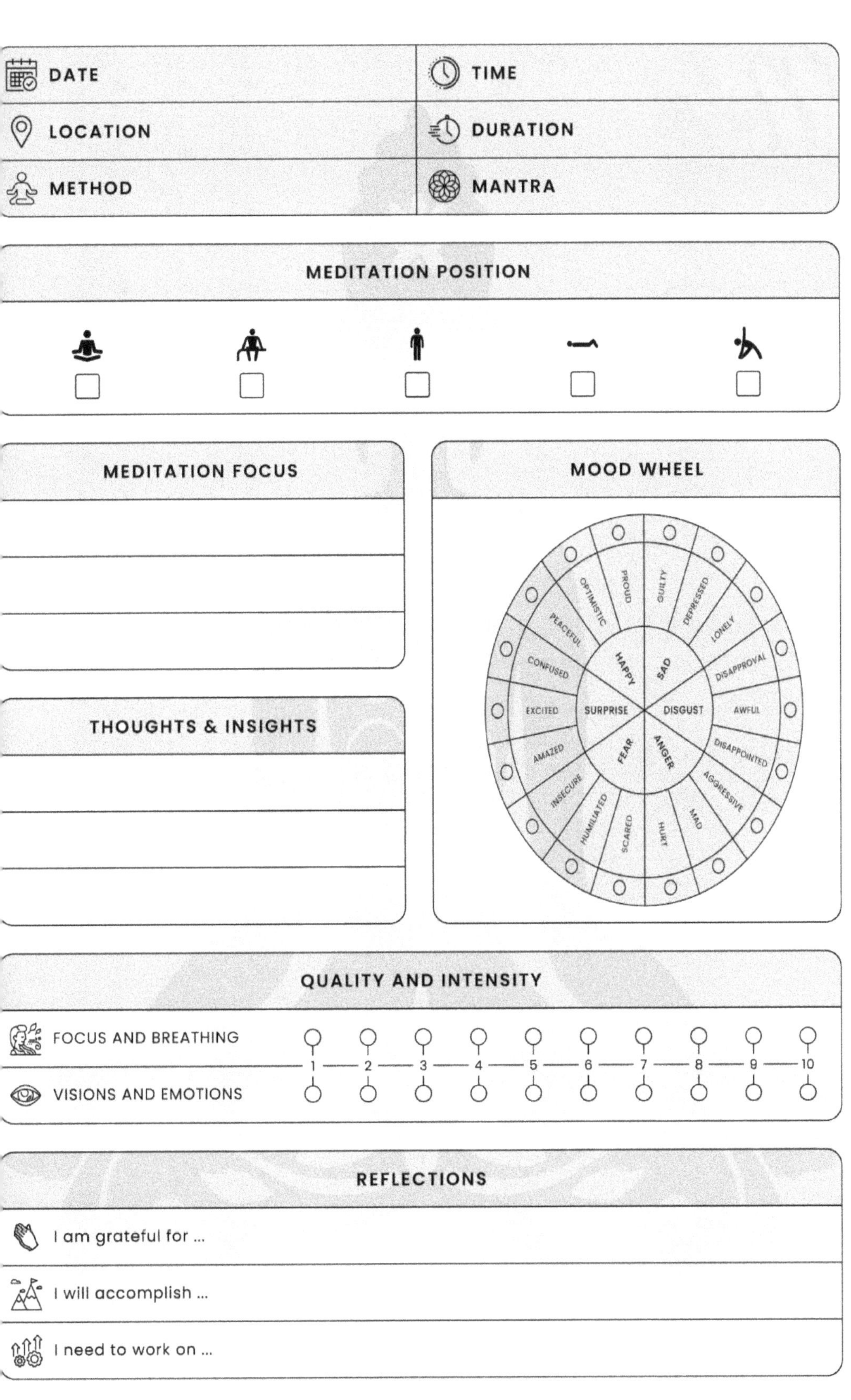DATE
TIME
LOCATION
DURATION
METHOD
MANTRA

MEDITATION POSITION

MEDITATION FOCUS

MOOD WHEEL

OPTIMISTIC
PROUD
GUILTY
DEPRESSED
PEACEFUL
LONELY
CONFUSED
HAPPY
SAD
DISAPPROVAL
EXCITED
SURPRISE
DISGUST
AWFUL
AMAZED
FEAR
ANGER
DISAPPOINTED
INSECURE
AGGRESSIVE
HUMILIATED
SCARED
HURT
MAD

THOUGHTS & INSIGHTS

QUALITY AND INTENSITY

FOCUS AND BREATHING
1 — 2 — 3 — 4 — 5 — 6 — 7 — 8 — 9 — 10
VISIONS AND EMOTIONS

REFLECTIONS

I am grateful for ...

I will accomplish ...

I need to work on ...

Notes

WHAT I LIKED

WHAT I DID NOT LIKE

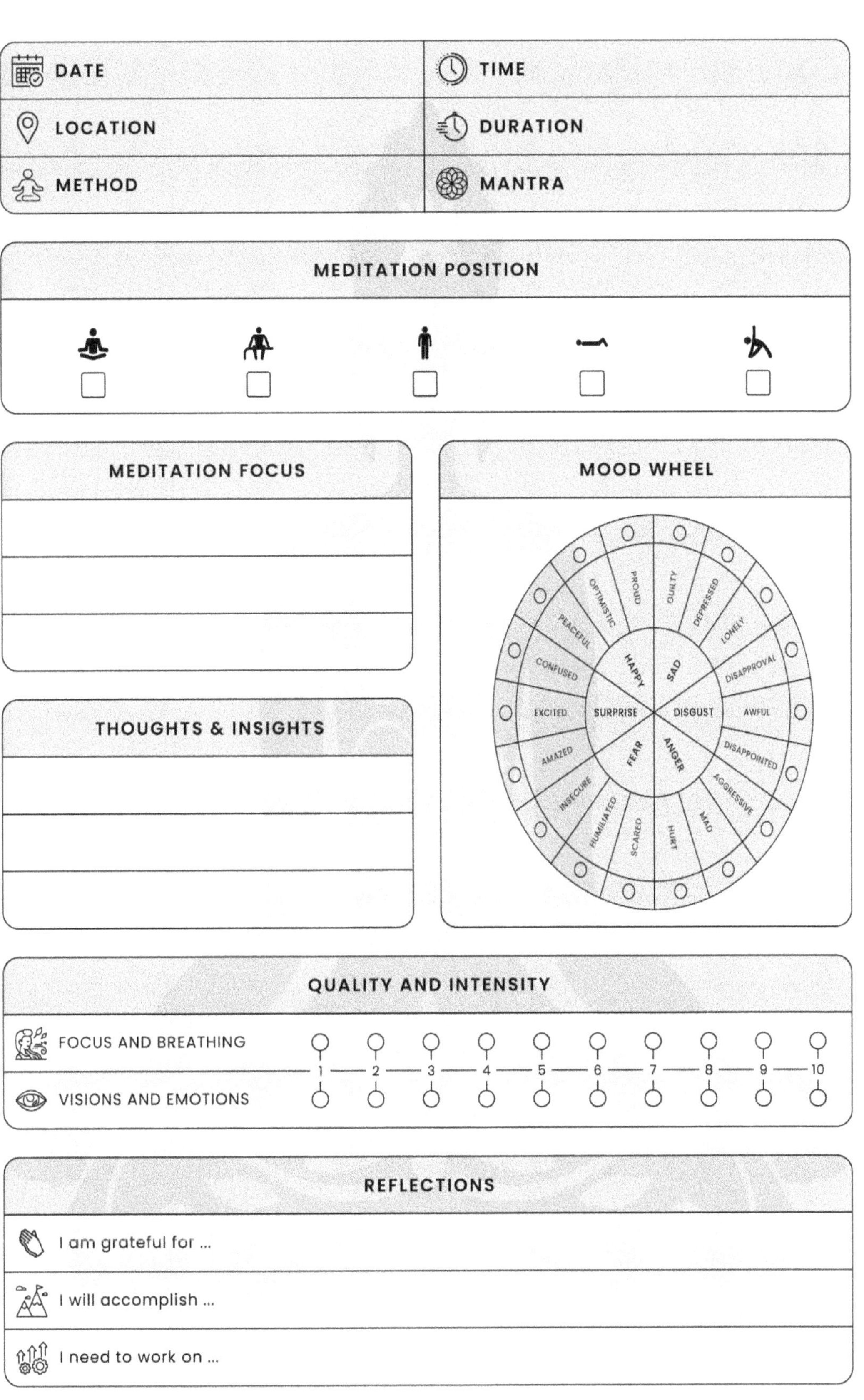

DATE
TIME
LOCATION
DURATION
METHOD
MANTRA
MEDITATION POSITION
MEDITATION FOCUS
MOOD WHEEL
OPTIMISTIC
PROUD
GUILTY
DEPRESSED
PEACEFUL
LONELY
CONFUSED
HAPPY
SAD
DISAPPROVAL
EXCITED
SURPRISE
DISGUST
AWFUL
AMAZED
FEAR
ANGER
DISAPPOINTED
INSECURE
AGGRESSIVE
HUMILIATED
SCARED
HURT
MAD
THOUGHTS & INSIGHTS
QUALITY AND INTENSITY
FOCUS AND BREATHING
1 2 3 4 5 6 7 8 9 10
VISIONS AND EMOTIONS
REFLECTIONS
I am grateful for ...
I will accomplish ...
I need to work on ...

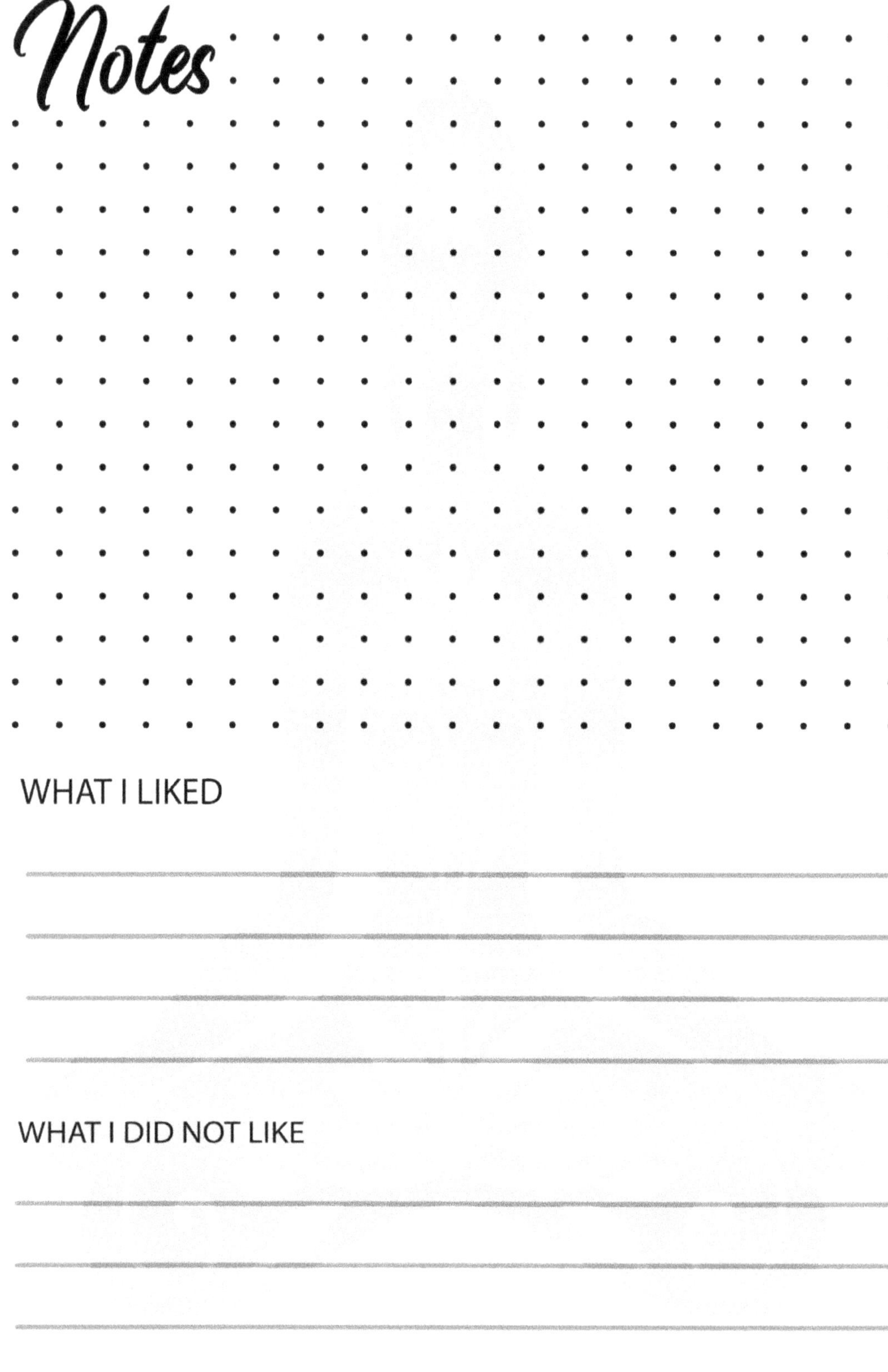

Notes

WHAT I LIKED

WHAT I DID NOT LIKE

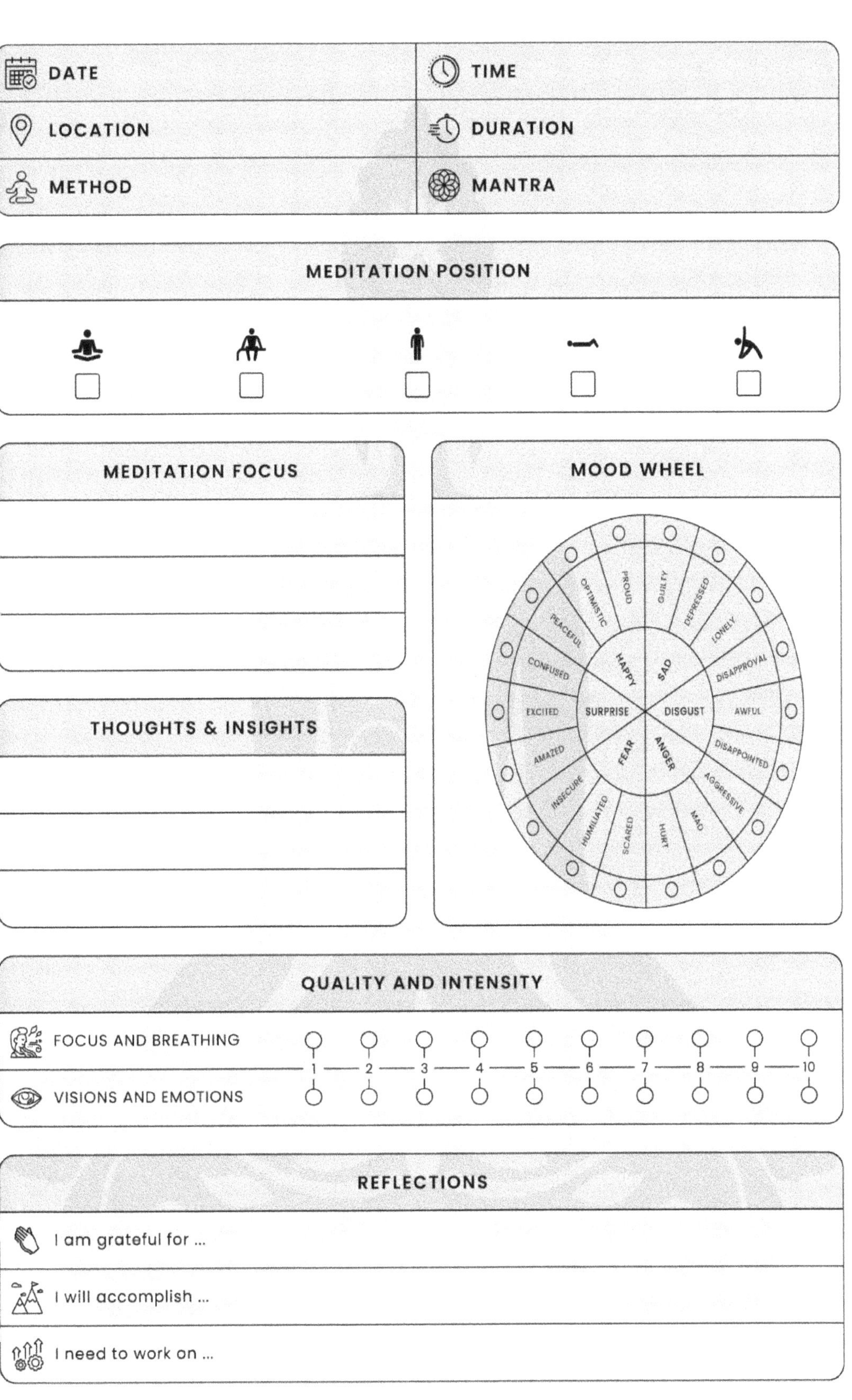

DATE
TIME
LOCATION
DURATION
METHOD
MANTRA

MEDITATION POSITION

MEDITATION FOCUS

MOOD WHEEL

OPTIMISTIC
PROUD
GUILTY
DEPRESSED
PEACEFUL
LONELY
CONFUSED
HAPPY
SAD
DISAPPROVAL
EXCITED
SURPRISE
DISGUST
AWFUL
AMAZED
FEAR
ANGER
DISAPPOINTED
INSECURE
AGGRESSIVE
HUMILIATED
SCARED
HURT
MAD

THOUGHTS & INSIGHTS

QUALITY AND INTENSITY

FOCUS AND BREATHING
1 — 2 — 3 — 4 — 5 — 6 — 7 — 8 — 9 — 10
VISIONS AND EMOTIONS

REFLECTIONS

I am grateful for ...

I will accomplish ...

I need to work on ...

Notes

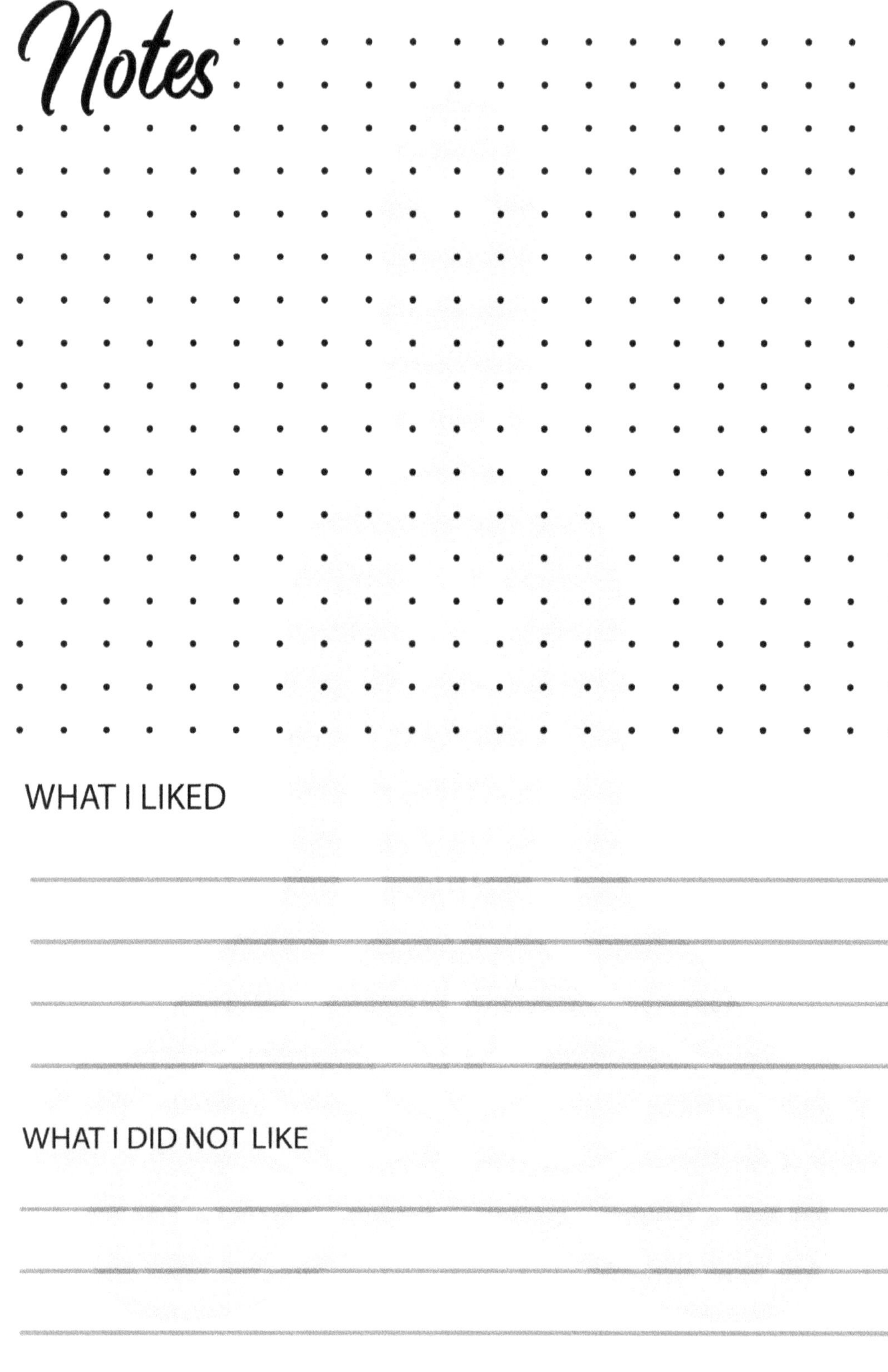

WHAT I LIKED

WHAT I DID NOT LIKE

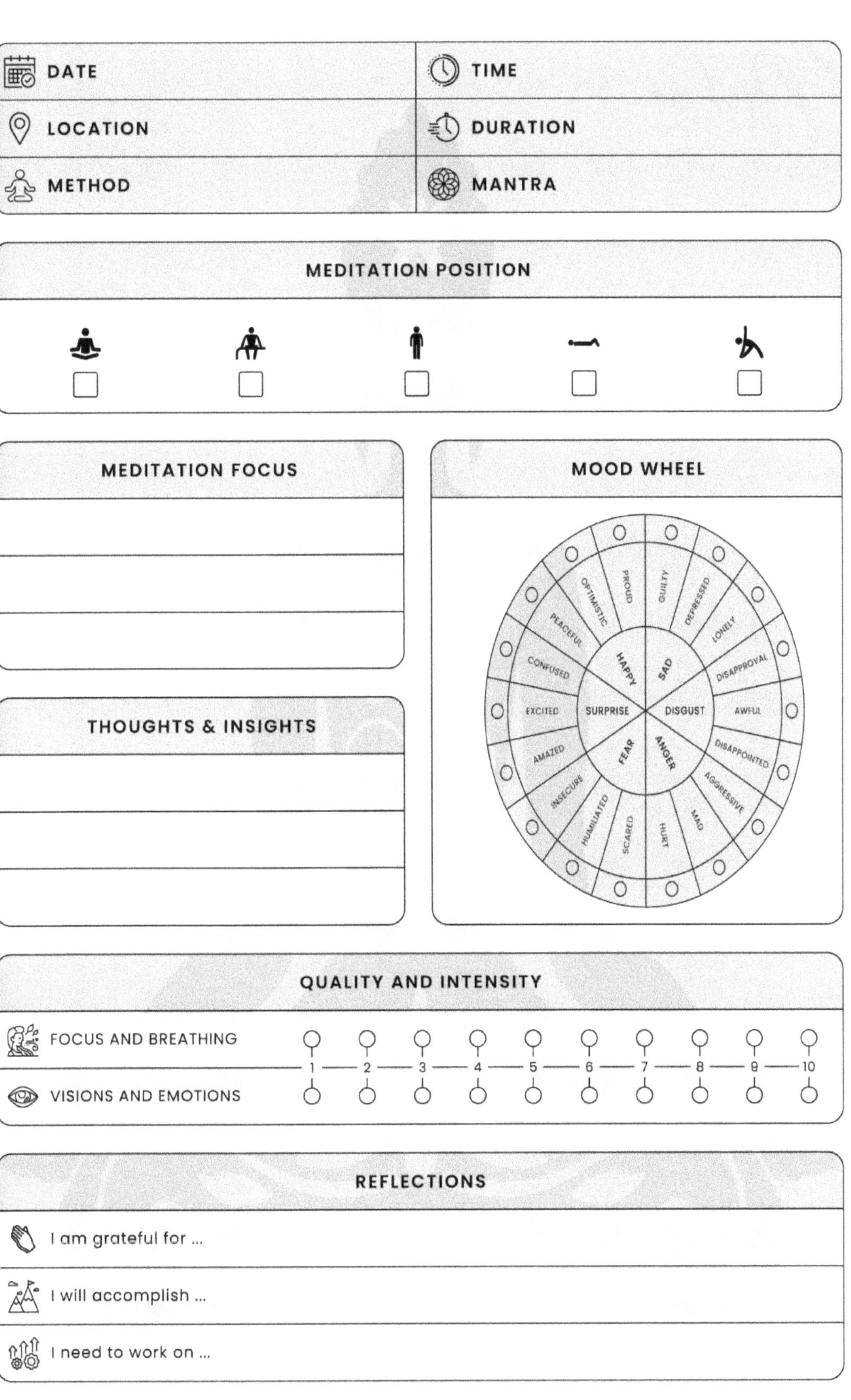

DATE
TIME
LOCATION
DURATION
METHOD
MANTRA

MEDITATION POSITION

MEDITATION FOCUS

MOOD WHEEL

OPTIMISTIC
PROUD
GUILTY
DEPRESSED
PEACEFUL
LONELY
CONFUSED
DISAPPROVAL
HAPPY
SAD
EXCITED
SURPRISE
DISGUST
AWFUL
AMAZED
DISAPPOINTED
FEAR
ANGER
INSECURE
AGGRESSIVE
HUMILIATED
SCARED
HURT
MAD

THOUGHTS & INSIGHTS

QUALITY AND INTENSITY

FOCUS AND BREATHING
1 — 2 — 3 — 4 — 5 — 6 — 7 — 8 — 9 — 10
VISIONS AND EMOTIONS

REFLECTIONS

I am grateful for ...
I will accomplish ...
I need to work on ...

Notes

WHAT I LIKED

WHAT I DID NOT LIKE

DATE	TIME
LOCATION	DURATION
METHOD	MANTRA

MEDITATION POSITION

☐ ☐ ☐ ☐ ☐

MEDITATION FOCUS

MOOD WHEEL

THOUGHTS & INSIGHTS

QUALITY AND INTENSITY

FOCUS AND BREATHING

1 — 2 — 3 — 4 — 5 — 6 — 7 — 8 — 9 — 10

VISIONS AND EMOTIONS

REFLECTIONS

I am grateful for ...

I will accomplish ...

I need to work on ...

Notes

WHAT I LIKED

WHAT I DID NOT LIKE

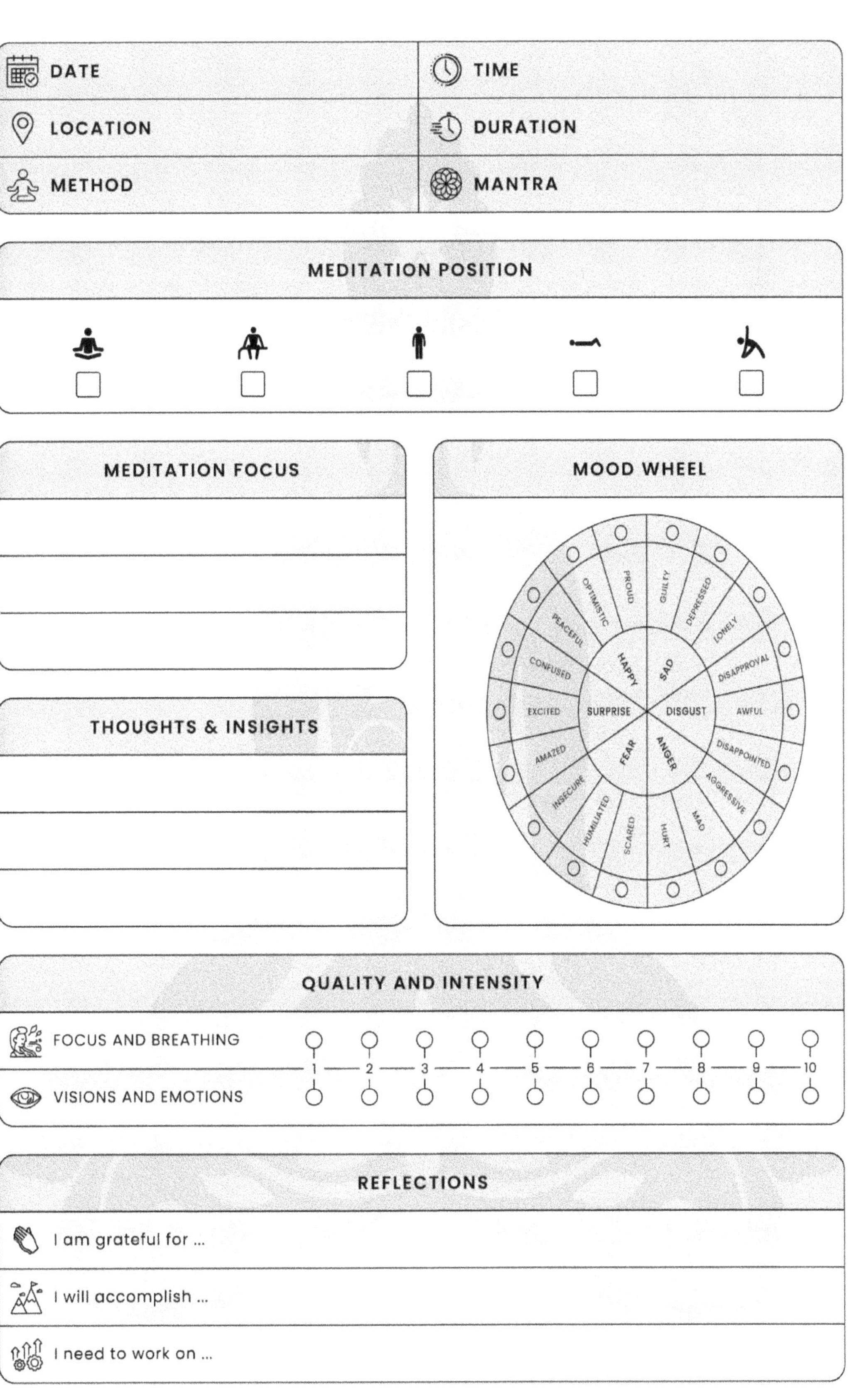

DATE	TIME
LOCATION	DURATION
METHOD	MANTRA

MEDITATION POSITION

☐ ☐ ☐ ☐ ☐

MEDITATION FOCUS

THOUGHTS & INSIGHTS

MOOD WHEEL

QUALITY AND INTENSITY

FOCUS AND BREATHING

1 — 2 — 3 — 4 — 5 — 6 — 7 — 8 — 9 — 10

VISIONS AND EMOTIONS

REFLECTIONS

I am grateful for ...

I will accomplish ...

I need to work on ...

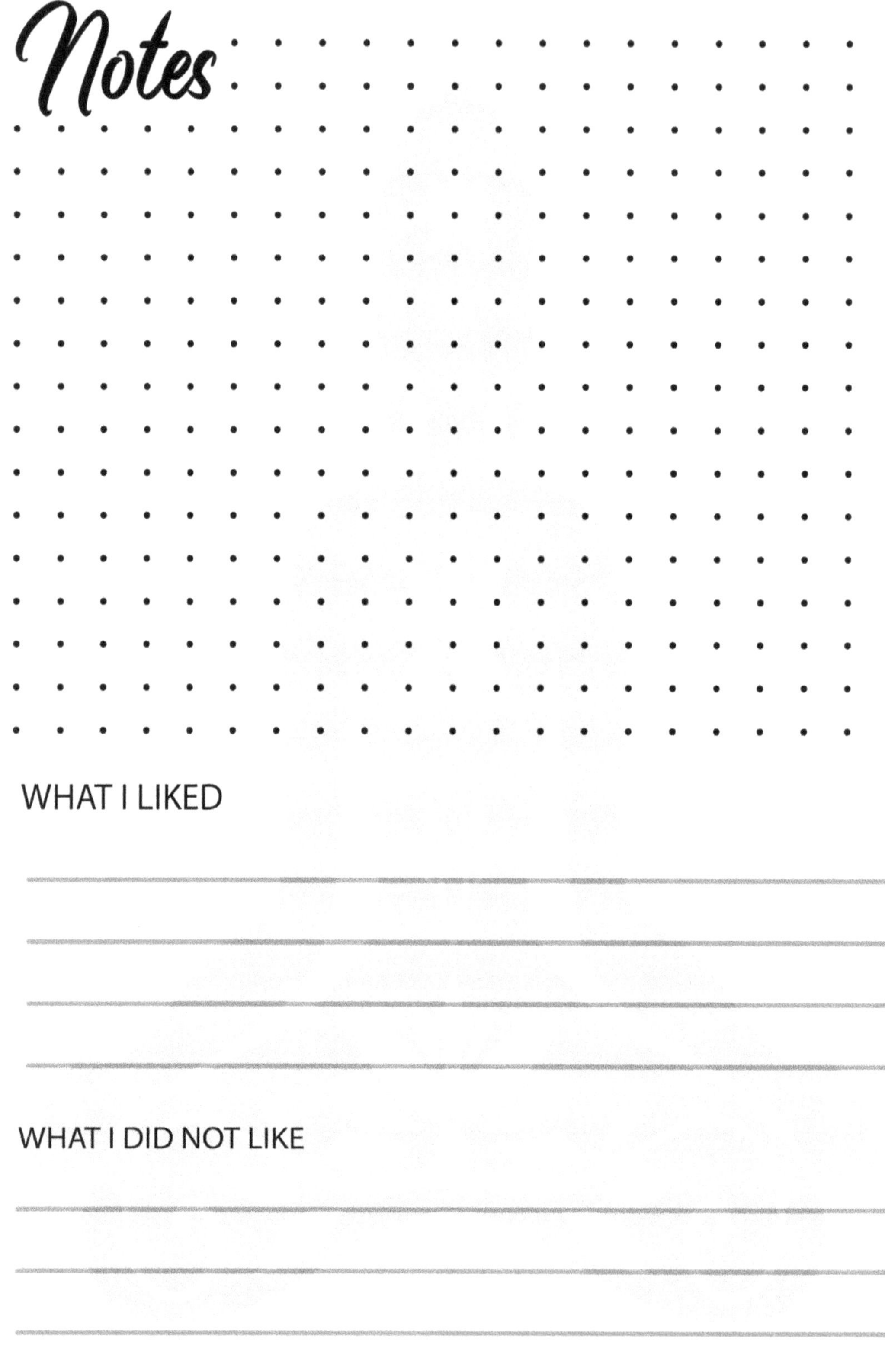

Notes

WHAT I LIKED

WHAT I DID NOT LIKE

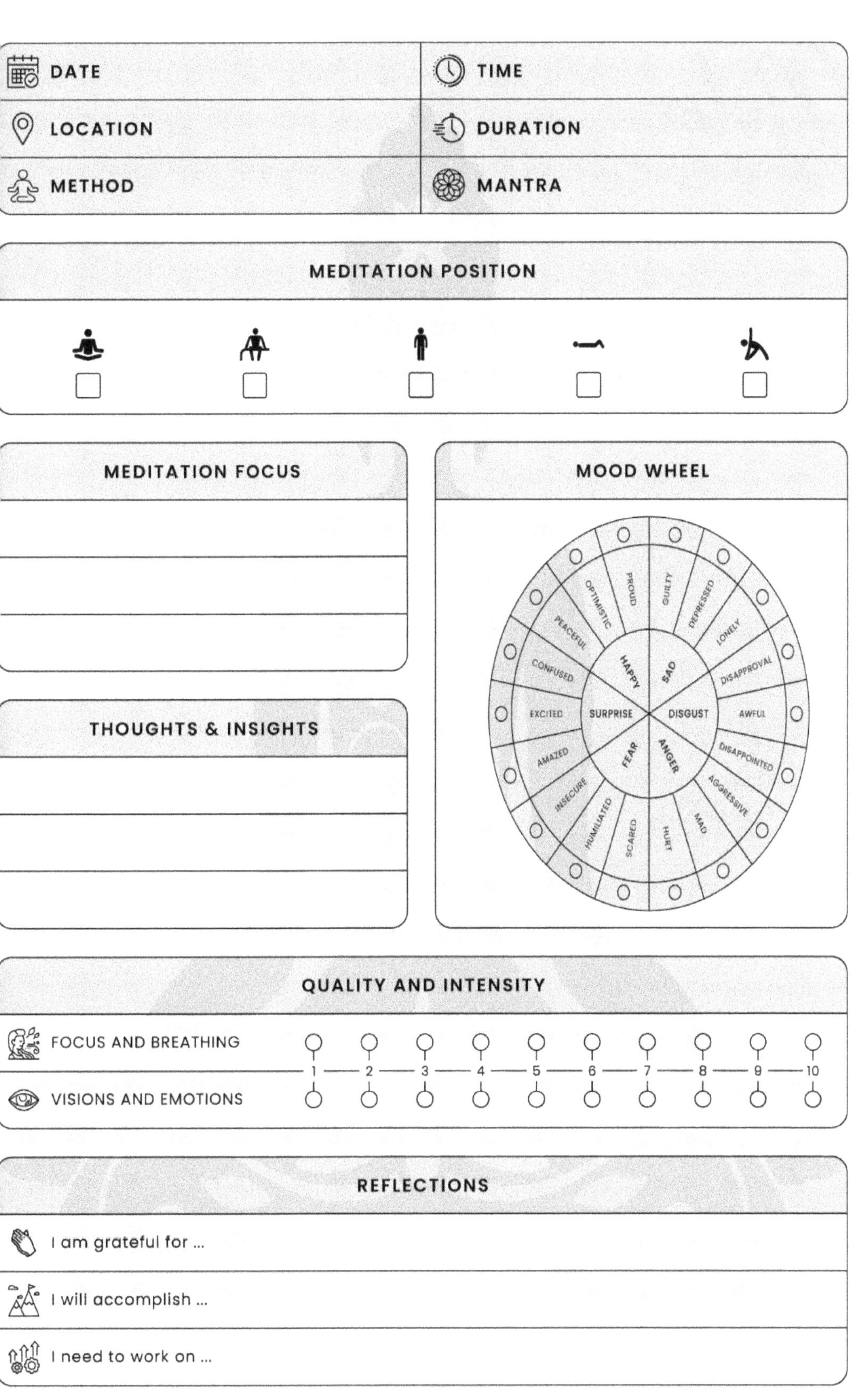
DATE
TIME
LOCATION
DURATION
METHOD
MANTRA
MEDITATION POSITION
MEDITATION FOCUS
MOOD WHEEL
OPTIMISTIC
PROUD
GUILTY
DEPRESSED
PEACEFUL
LONELY
CONFUSED
HAPPY
SAD
DISAPPROVAL
EXCITED
SURPRISE
DISGUST
AWFUL
AMAZED
FEAR
ANGER
DISAPPOINTED
INSECURE
AGGRESSIVE
HUMILIATED
SCARED
HURT
MAD
THOUGHTS & INSIGHTS
QUALITY AND INTENSITY
FOCUS AND BREATHING
1 — 2 — 3 — 4 — 5 — 6 — 7 — 8 — 9 — 10
VISIONS AND EMOTIONS
REFLECTIONS
I am grateful for ...
I will accomplish ...
I need to work on ...

Notes

WHAT I LIKED

WHAT I DID NOT LIKE

<table>
<tr><td>📅 DATE</td><td>🕐 TIME</td></tr>
<tr><td>📍 LOCATION</td><td>⏱ DURATION</td></tr>
<tr><td>🧘 METHOD</td><td>✿ MANTRA</td></tr>
</table>

MEDITATION POSITION

☐   ☐   ☐   ☐   ☐

MEDITATION FOCUS

MOOD WHEEL

THOUGHTS & INSIGHTS

QUALITY AND INTENSITY

🌿 FOCUS AND BREATHING

1 — 2 — 3 — 4 — 5 — 6 — 7 — 8 — 9 — 10

👁 VISIONS AND EMOTIONS

REFLECTIONS

✍ I am grateful for ...

⛰ I will accomplish ...

⚙ I need to work on ...

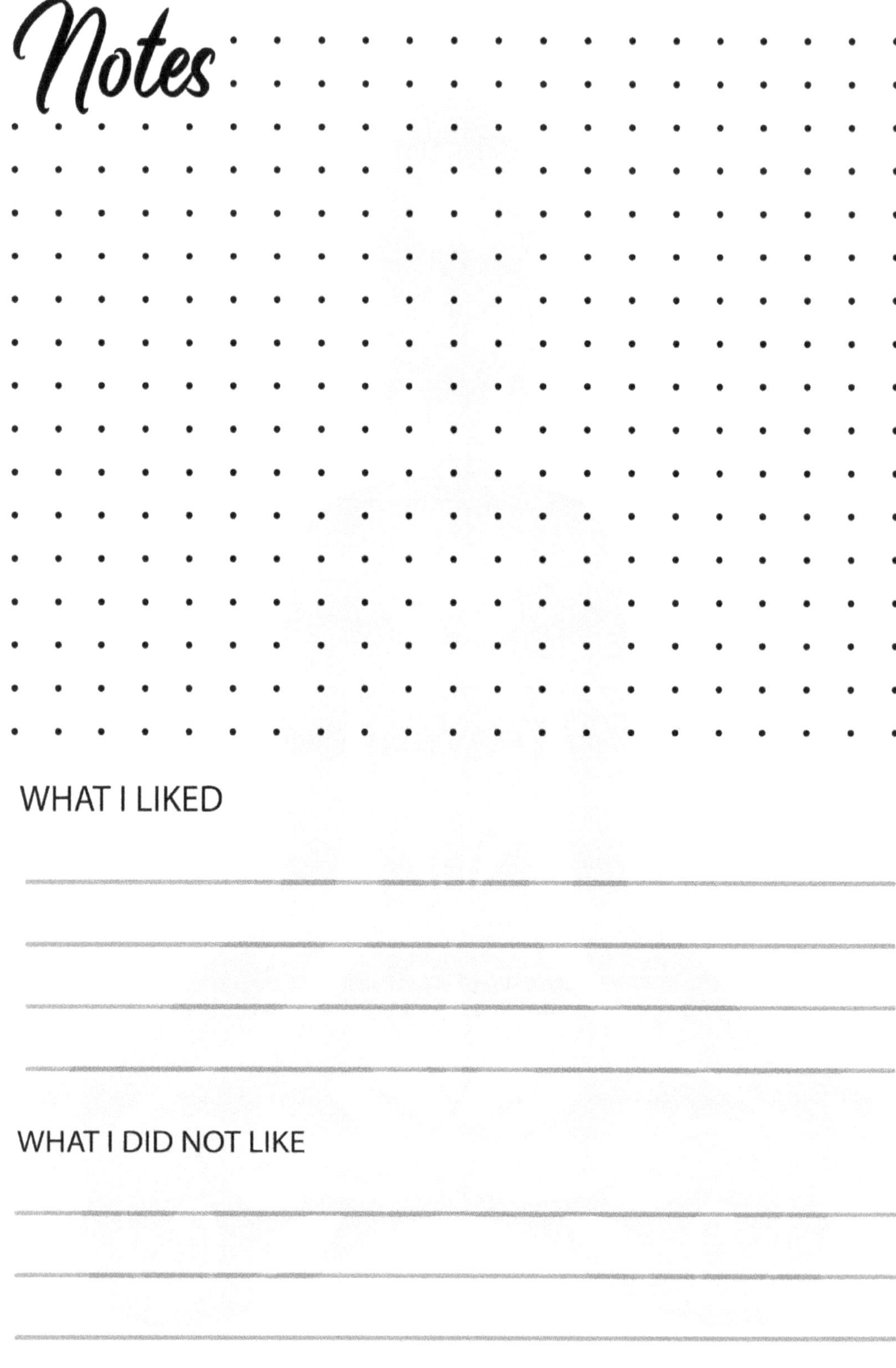

Notes

WHAT I LIKED

WHAT I DID NOT LIKE

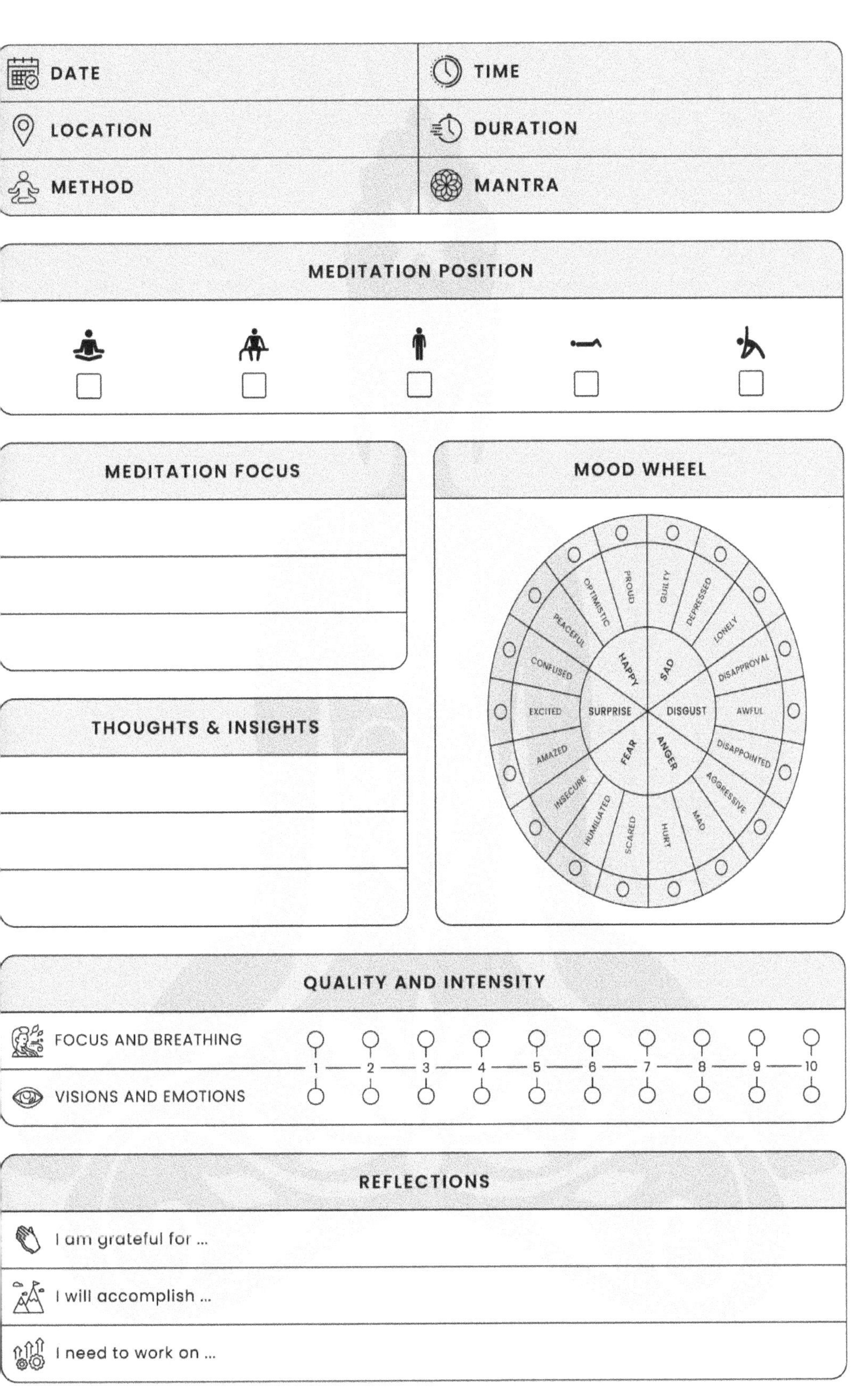

DATE
TIME
LOCATION
DURATION
METHOD
MANTRA
MEDITATION POSITION
MEDITATION FOCUS
MOOD WHEEL
OPTIMISTIC
PROUD
GUILTY
DEPRESSED
PEACEFUL
LONELY
CONFUSED
HAPPY
SAD
DISAPPROVAL
EXCITED
SURPRISE
DISGUST
AWFUL
AMAZED
FEAR
ANGER
DISAPPOINTED
INSECURE
AGGRESSIVE
HUMILIATED
SCARED
HURT
MAD
THOUGHTS & INSIGHTS
QUALITY AND INTENSITY
FOCUS AND BREATHING
1 — 2 — 3 — 4 — 5 — 6 — 7 — 8 — 9 — 10
VISIONS AND EMOTIONS
REFLECTIONS
I am grateful for ...
I will accomplish ...
I need to work on ...

Notes

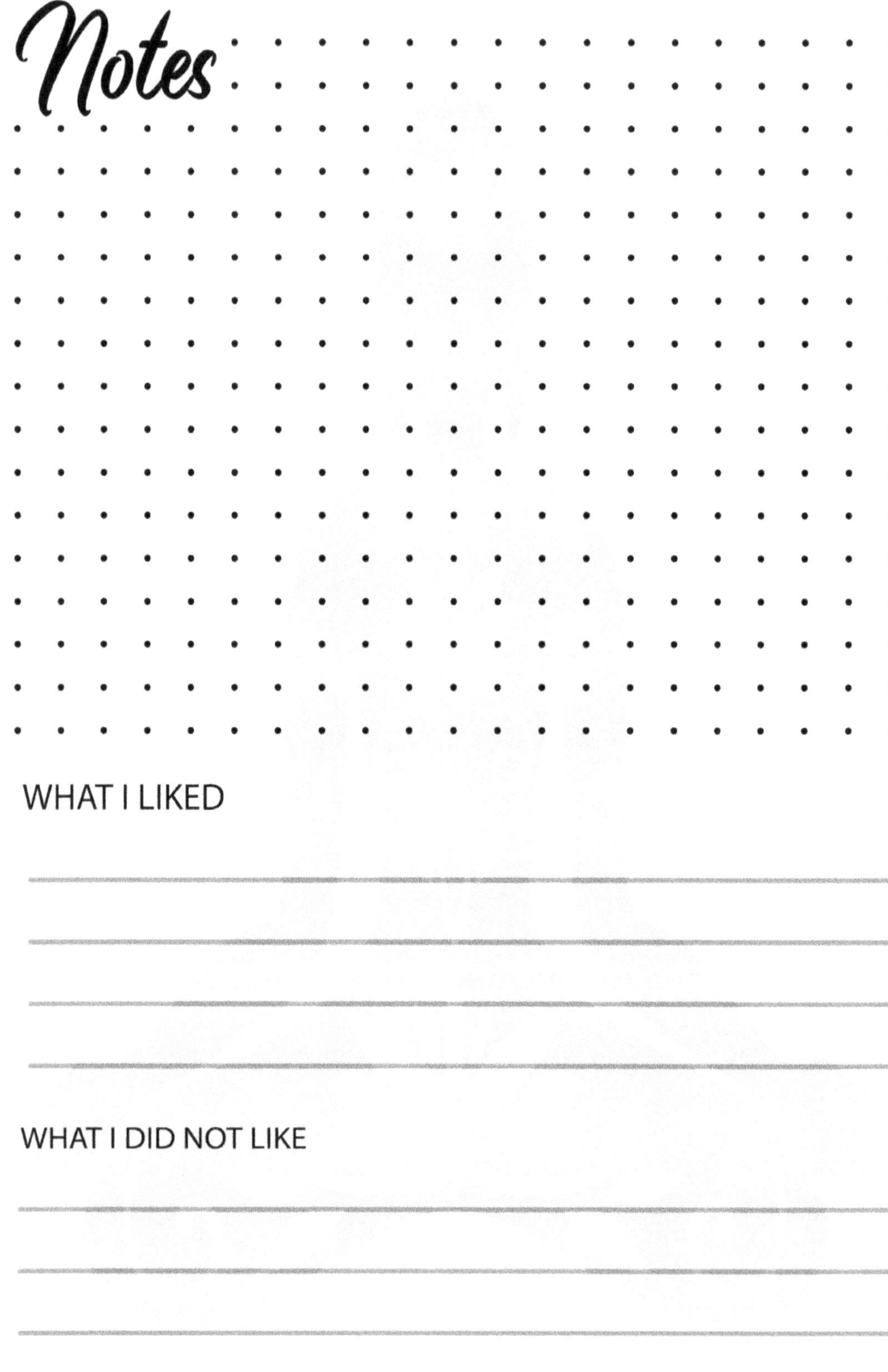

WHAT I LIKED

WHAT I DID NOT LIKE

MEDITATION JOURNAL

DATE	TIME
LOCATION	DURATION
METHOD	MANTRA

MEDITATION POSITION

☐ ☐ ☐ ☐ ☐

MEDITATION FOCUS

THOUGHTS & INSIGHTS

MOOD WHEEL

QUALITY AND INTENSITY

FOCUS AND BREATHING

1 — 2 — 3 — 4 — 5 — 6 — 7 — 8 — 9 — 10

VISIONS AND EMOTIONS

REFLECTIONS

I am grateful for ...

I will accomplish ...

I need to work on ...

Notes

WHAT I LIKED

WHAT I DID NOT LIKE

MEDITATION POSITION

MEDITATION FOCUS

THOUGHTS & INSIGHTS

MOOD WHEEL

QUALITY AND INTENSITY

REFLECTIONS

I am grateful for ...

I will accomplish ...

I need to work on ...

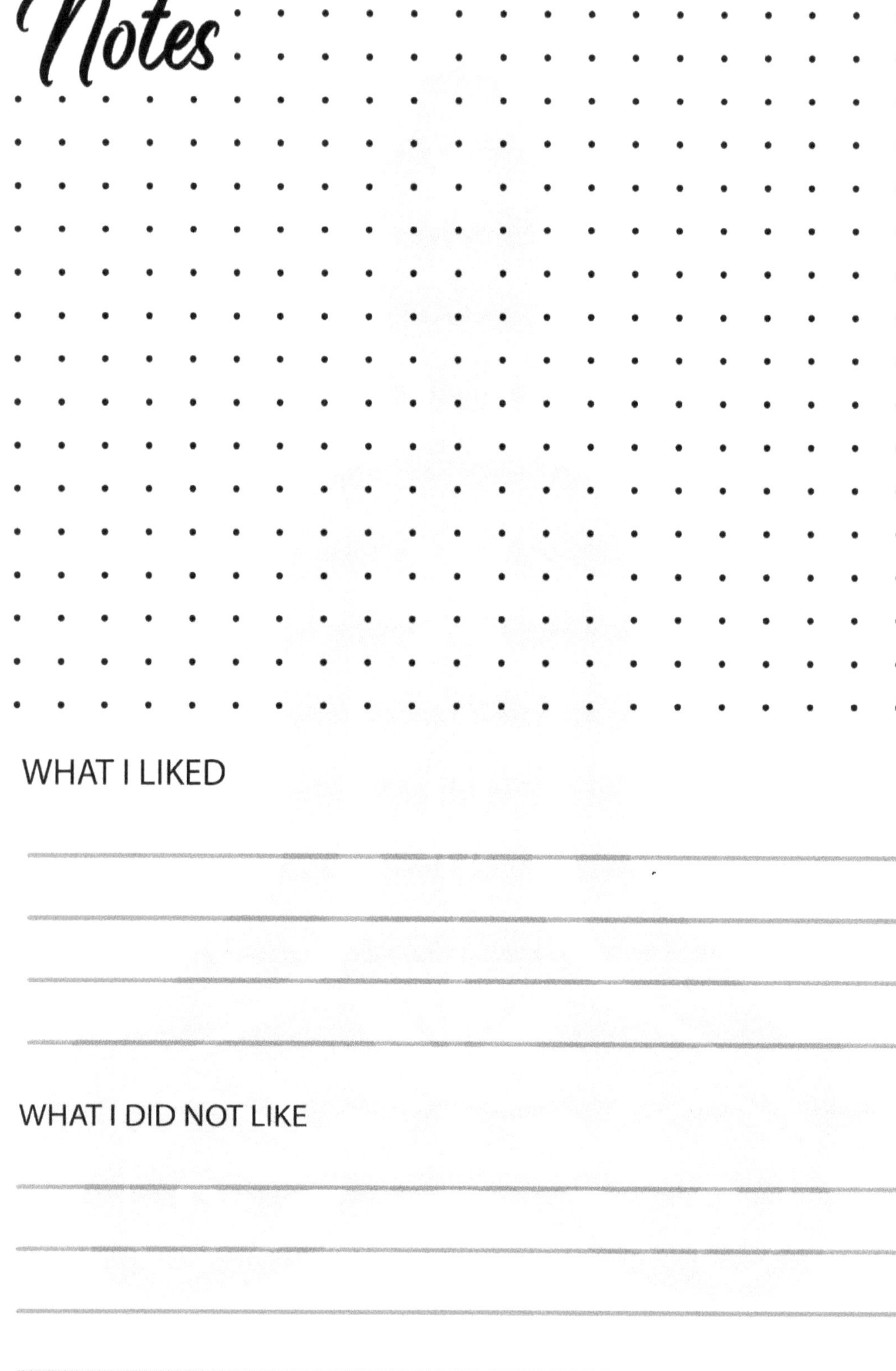

Notes
WHAT I LIKED
WHAT I DID NOT LIKE

MEDITATION POSITION

MEDITATION FOCUS

MOOD WHEEL

THOUGHTS & INSIGHTS

QUALITY AND INTENSITY

FOCUS AND BREATHING

1 — 2 — 3 — 4 — 5 — 6 — 7 — 8 — 9 — 10

VISIONS AND EMOTIONS

REFLECTIONS

I am grateful for ...

I will accomplish ...

I need to work on ...

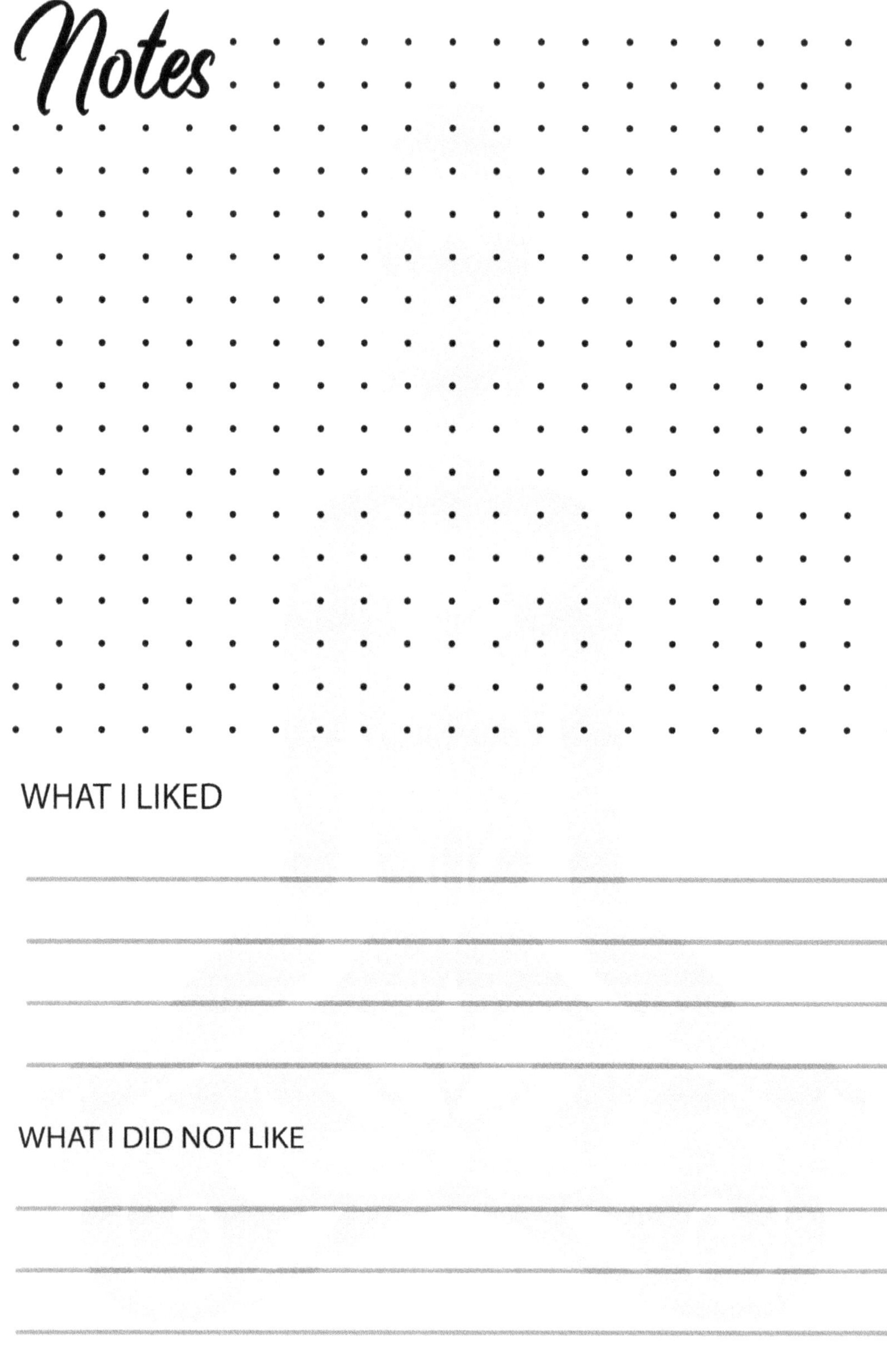

Notes

WHAT I LIKED

WHAT I DID NOT LIKE

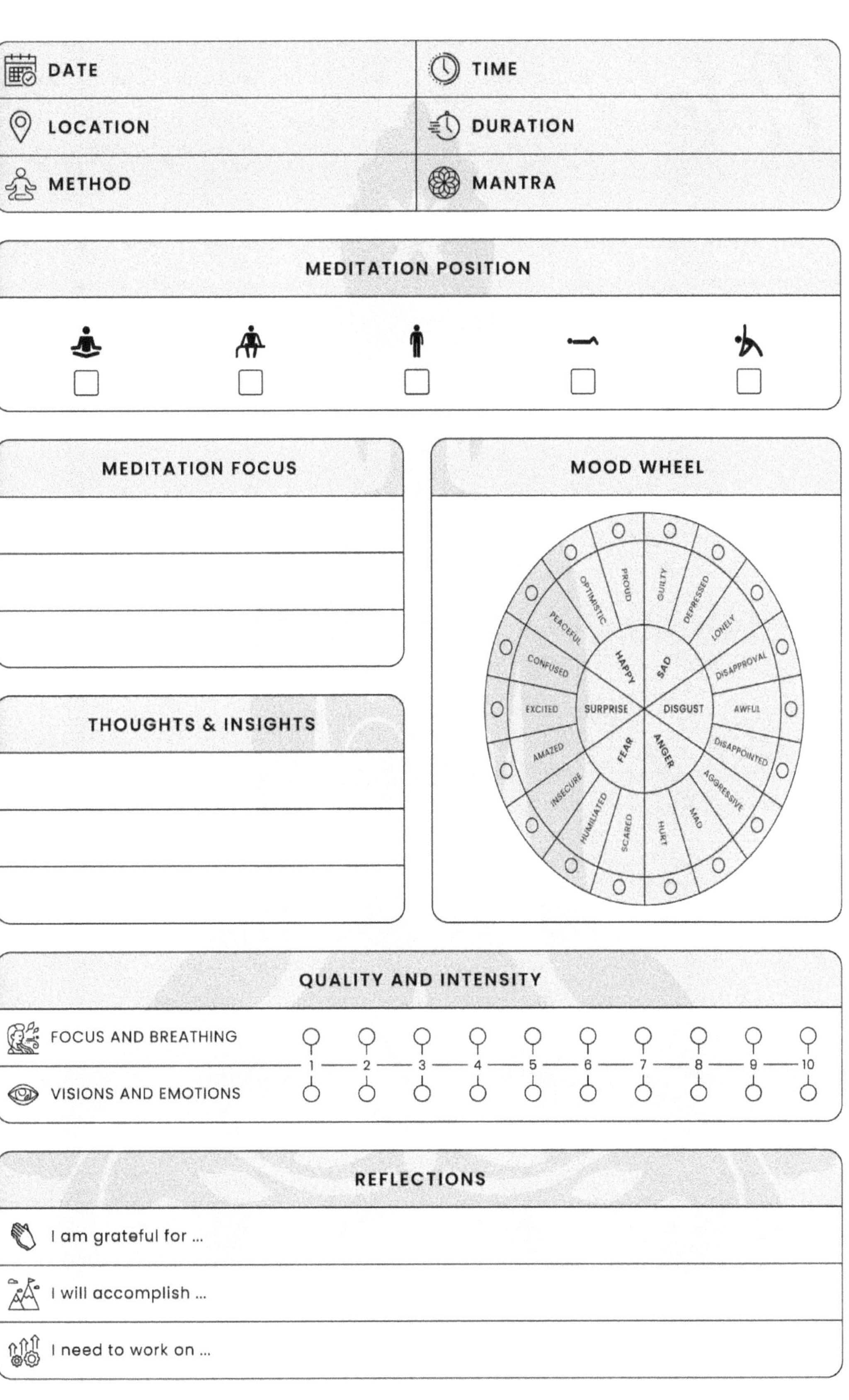

DATE
TIME
LOCATION
DURATION
METHOD
MANTRA

MEDITATION POSITION

MEDITATION FOCUS

MOOD WHEEL

OPTIMISTIC
PROUD
GUILTY
DEPRESSED
PEACEFUL
LONELY
CONFUSED
HAPPY
SAD
DISAPPROVAL
EXCITED
SURPRISE
DISGUST
AWFUL
AMAZED
FEAR
ANGER
DISAPPOINTED
INSECURE
AGGRESSIVE
HUMILIATED
SCARED
HURT
MAD

THOUGHTS & INSIGHTS

QUALITY AND INTENSITY

FOCUS AND BREATHING
1 2 3 4 5 6 7 8 9 10
VISIONS AND EMOTIONS

REFLECTIONS

I am grateful for ...

I will accomplish ...

I need to work on ...

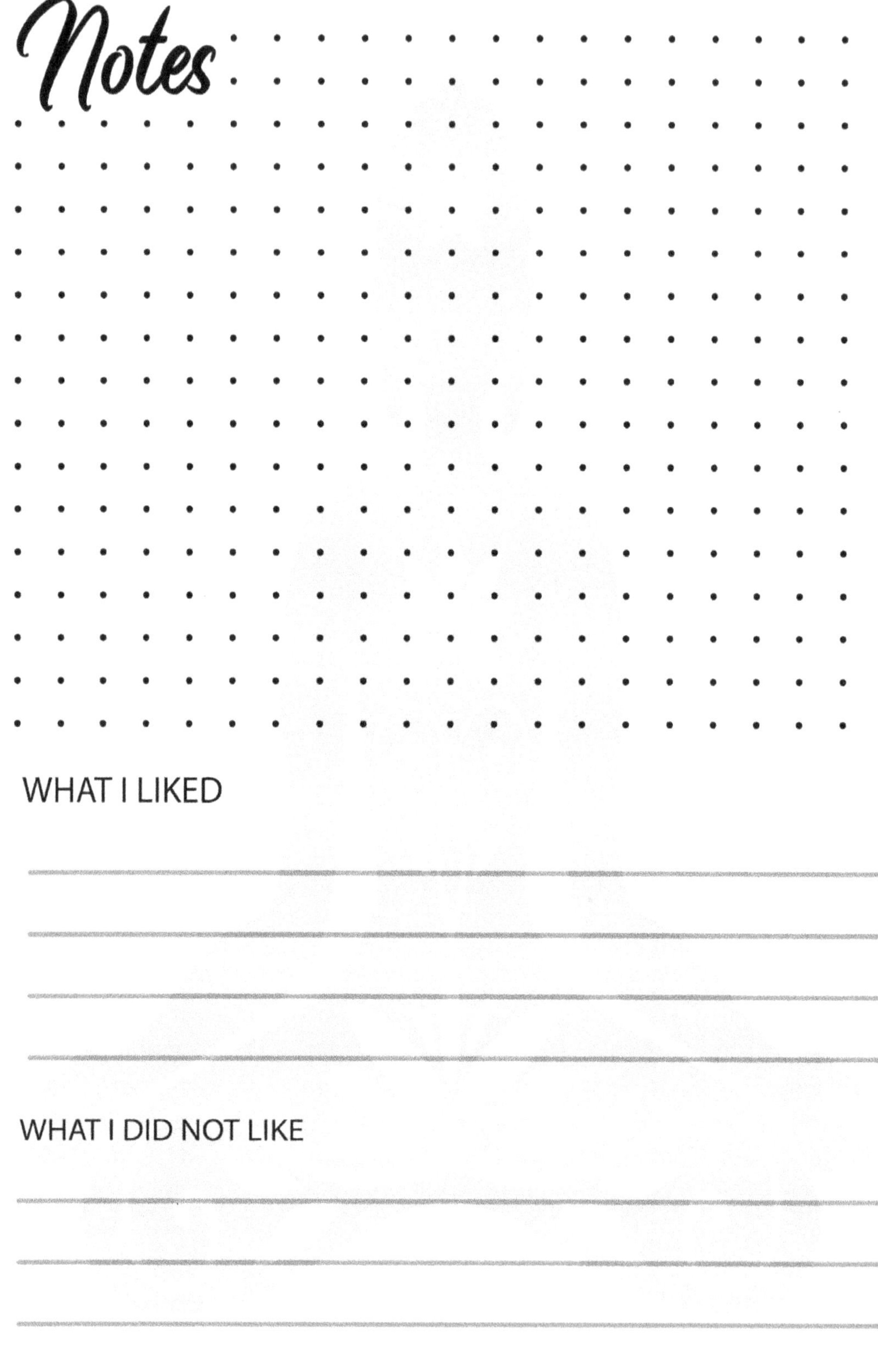

Notes

WHAT I LIKED

WHAT I DID NOT LIKE

📅 DATE	🕐 TIME
📍 LOCATION	⏱ DURATION
🧘 METHOD	✾ MANTRA

MEDITATION POSITION

☐ ☐ ☐ ☐ ☐

MEDITATION FOCUS

MOOD WHEEL

THOUGHTS & INSIGHTS

QUALITY AND INTENSITY

FOCUS AND BREATHING

1 — 2 — 3 — 4 — 5 — 6 — 7 — 8 — 9 — 10

VISIONS AND EMOTIONS

REFLECTIONS

I am grateful for ...

I will accomplish ...

I need to work on ...

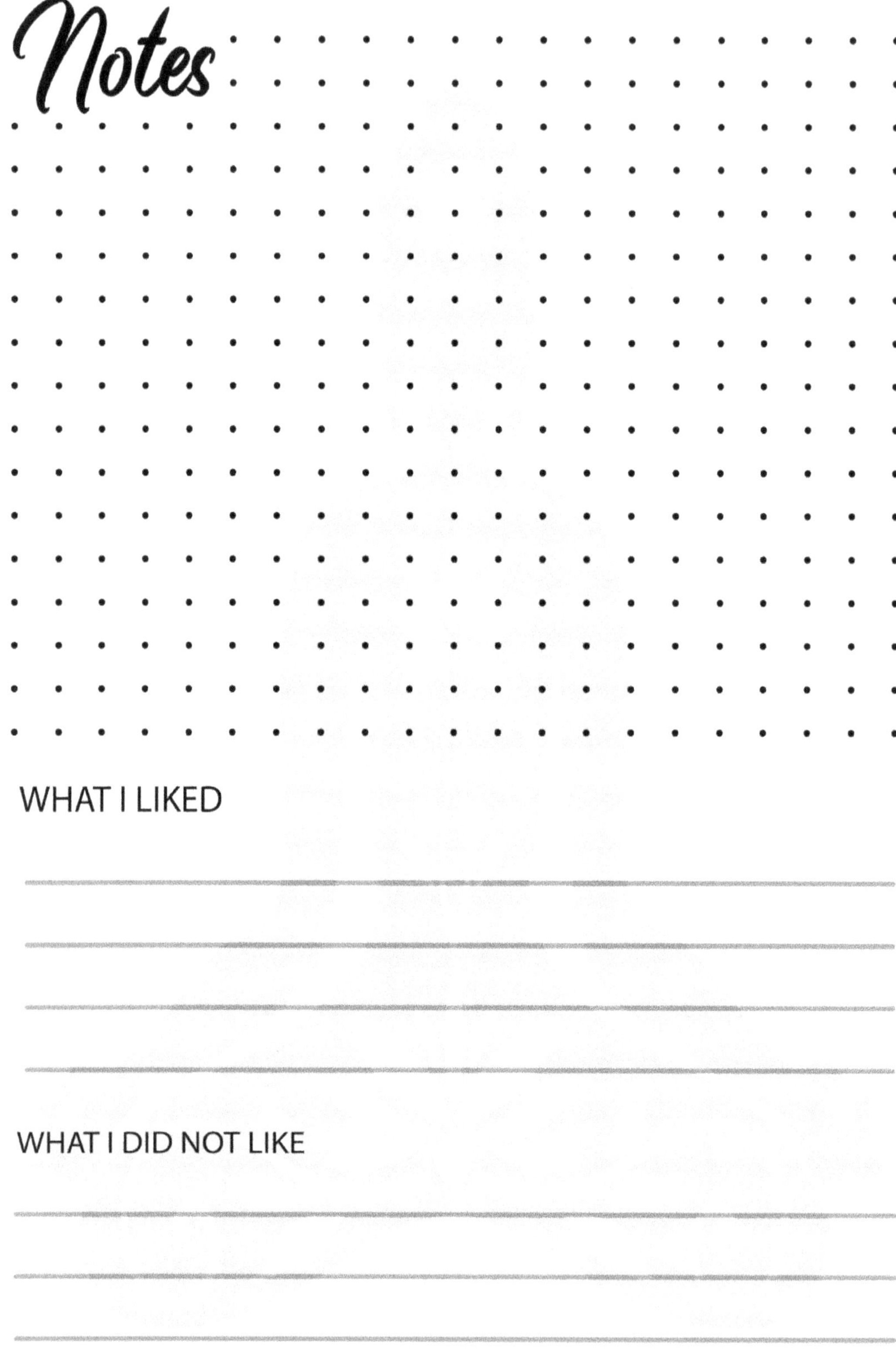

Notes

WHAT I LIKED

WHAT I DID NOT LIKE

DATE		TIME
LOCATION		DURATION
METHOD		MANTRA

MEDITATION POSITION

MEDITATION FOCUS

MOOD WHEEL

THOUGHTS & INSIGHTS

QUALITY AND INTENSITY

FOCUS AND BREATHING

1 — 2 — 3 — 4 — 5 — 6 — 7 — 8 — 9 — 10

VISIONS AND EMOTIONS

REFLECTIONS

I am grateful for ...

I will accomplish ...

I need to work on ...

Notes

WHAT I LIKED

WHAT I DID NOT LIKE

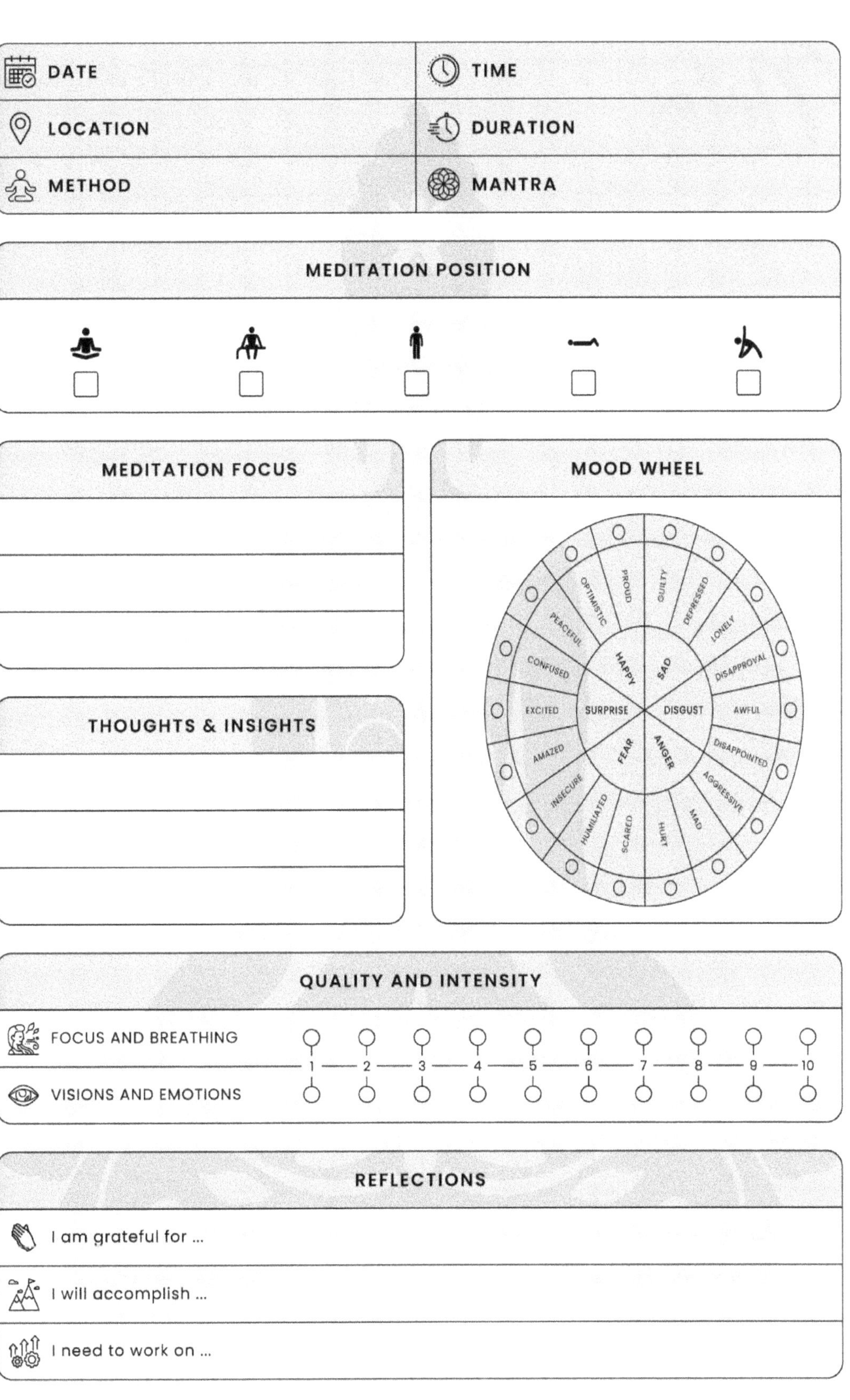

DATE
TIME
LOCATION
DURATION
METHOD
MANTRA

MEDITATION POSITION

MEDITATION FOCUS

MOOD WHEEL

OPTIMISTIC
PROUD
GUILTY
DEPRESSED
PLACEFUL
LONELY
CONFUSED
HAPPY
SAD
DISAPPROVAL
EXCITED
SURPRISE
DISGUST
AWFUL
AMAZED
FEAR
ANGER
DISAPPOINTED
INSECURE
AGGRESSIVE
HUMILIATED
SCARED
HURT
MAD

THOUGHTS & INSIGHTS

QUALITY AND INTENSITY

FOCUS AND BREATHING
1 — 2 — 3 — 4 — 5 — 6 — 7 — 8 — 9 — 10
VISIONS AND EMOTIONS

REFLECTIONS

I am grateful for ...

I will accomplish ...

I need to work on ...

Notes

WHAT I LIKED

WHAT I DID NOT LIKE

<table>
<tr><td>📅 DATE</td><td>🕐 TIME</td></tr>
<tr><td>📍 LOCATION</td><td>⏱ DURATION</td></tr>
<tr><td>🧘 METHOD</td><td>❀ MANTRA</td></tr>
</table>

MEDITATION POSITION

☐ ☐ ☐ ☐ ☐

MEDITATION FOCUS

THOUGHTS & INSIGHTS

MOOD WHEEL

QUALITY AND INTENSITY

🧠 FOCUS AND BREATHING

1 — 2 — 3 — 4 — 5 — 6 — 7 — 8 — 9 — 10

👁 VISIONS AND EMOTIONS

REFLECTIONS

I am grateful for ...

I will accomplish ...

I need to work on ...

Notes

WHAT I LIKED

WHAT I DID NOT LIKE

DATE

TIME

LOCATION

DURATION

METHOD

MANTRA

MEDITATION POSITION

☐ ☐ ☐ ☐ ☐

MEDITATION FOCUS

MOOD WHEEL

THOUGHTS & INSIGHTS

QUALITY AND INTENSITY

FOCUS AND BREATHING

1 — 2 — 3 — 4 — 5 — 6 — 7 — 8 — 9 — 10

VISIONS AND EMOTIONS

REFLECTIONS

I am grateful for ...

I will accomplish ...

I need to work on ...

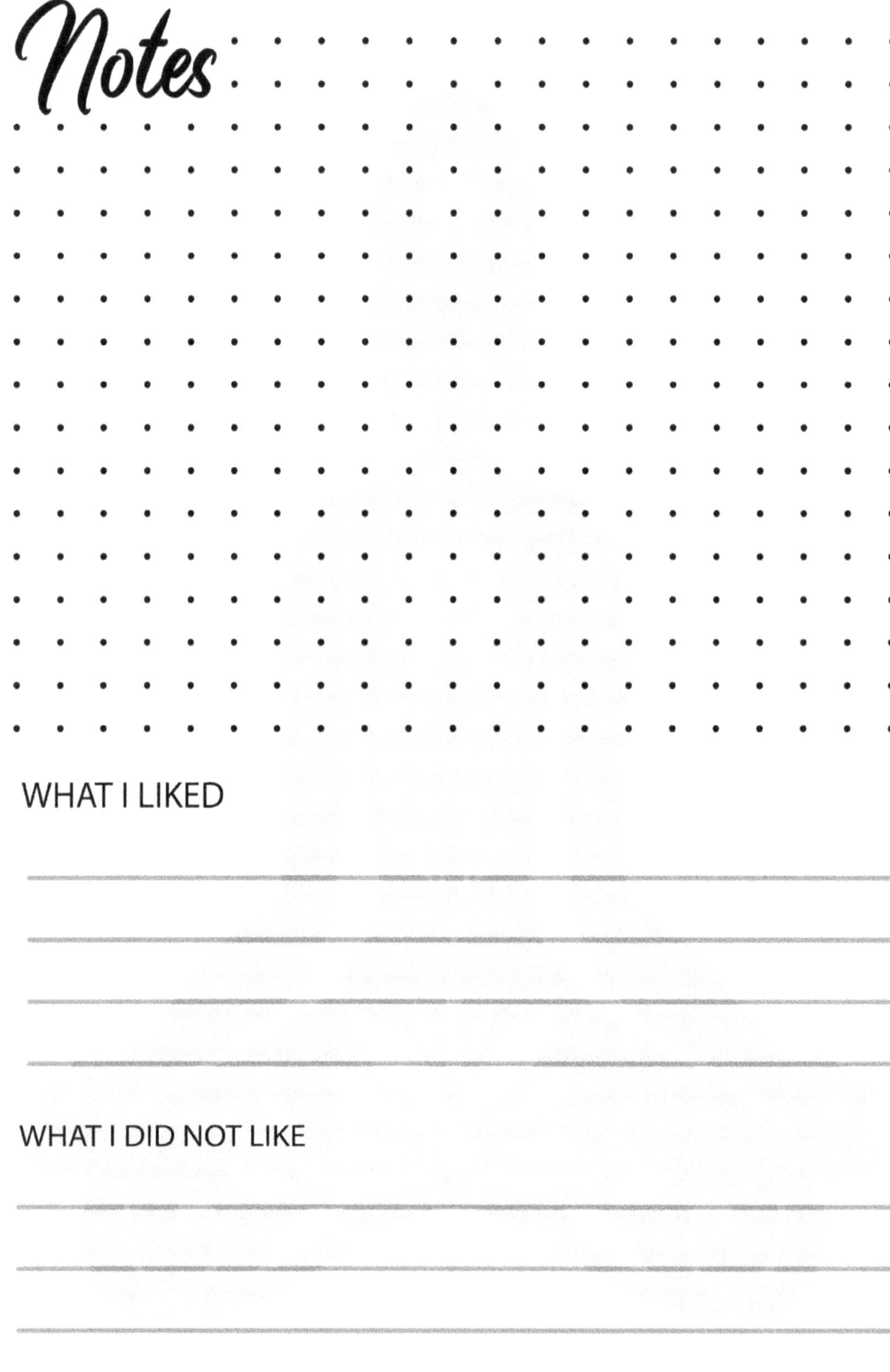

Notes

WHAT I LIKED

WHAT I DID NOT LIKE

<table>
<tr><td>DATE</td><td>TIME</td></tr>
<tr><td>LOCATION</td><td>DURATION</td></tr>
<tr><td>METHOD</td><td>MANTRA</td></tr>
</table>

MEDITATION POSITION

MEDITATION FOCUS

MOOD WHEEL

THOUGHTS & INSIGHTS

QUALITY AND INTENSITY

FOCUS AND BREATHING

1 — 2 — 3 — 4 — 5 — 6 — 7 — 8 — 9 — 10

VISIONS AND EMOTIONS

REFLECTIONS

I am grateful for ...

I will accomplish ...

I need to work on ...

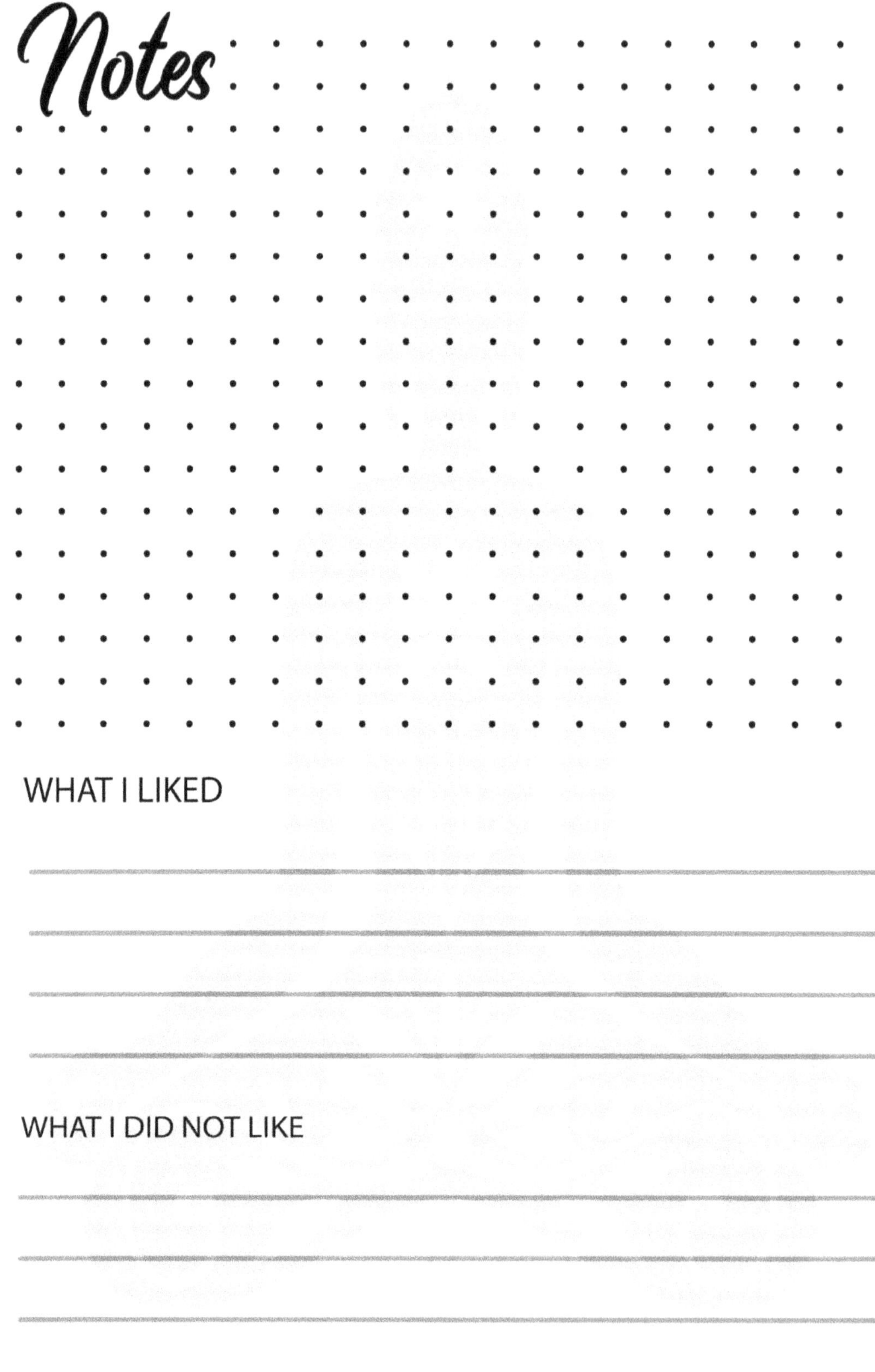

Notes

WHAT I LIKED

WHAT I DID NOT LIKE

MEDITATION POSITION

DATE	TIME
LOCATION	DURATION
METHOD	MANTRA

MEDITATION POSITION

MEDITATION FOCUS

THOUGHTS & INSIGHTS

MOOD WHEEL

QUALITY AND INTENSITY

FOCUS AND BREATHING

1 — 2 — 3 — 4 — 5 — 6 — 7 — 8 — 9 — 10

VISIONS AND EMOTIONS

REFLECTIONS

I am grateful for ...

I will accomplish ...

I need to work on ...

Notes

WHAT I LIKED

WHAT I DID NOT LIKE

MEDITATION POSITION

MEDITATION FOCUS

THOUGHTS & INSIGHTS

MOOD WHEEL

QUALITY AND INTENSITY

FOCUS AND BREATHING

1 — 2 — 3 — 4 — 5 — 6 — 7 — 8 — 9 — 10

VISIONS AND EMOTIONS

REFLECTIONS

I am grateful for ...

I will accomplish ...

I need to work on ...

Notes

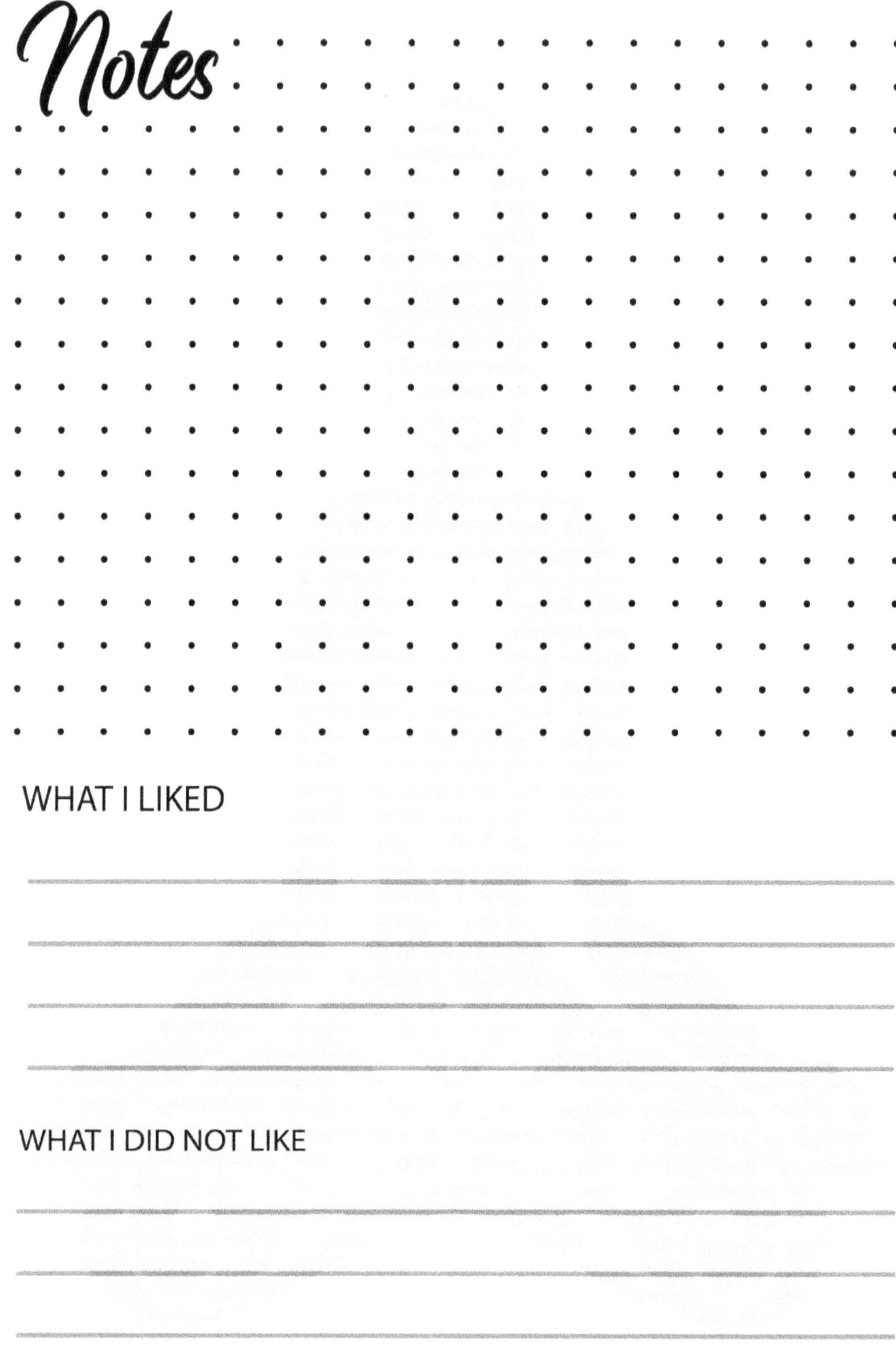

WHAT I LIKED

WHAT I DID NOT LIKE